Behavioral Pharmacology - From Basic to Clinical Research

Edited by Juan Francisco Rodríguez-Landa and Jonathan Cueto-Escobedo

Published in London, United Kingdom

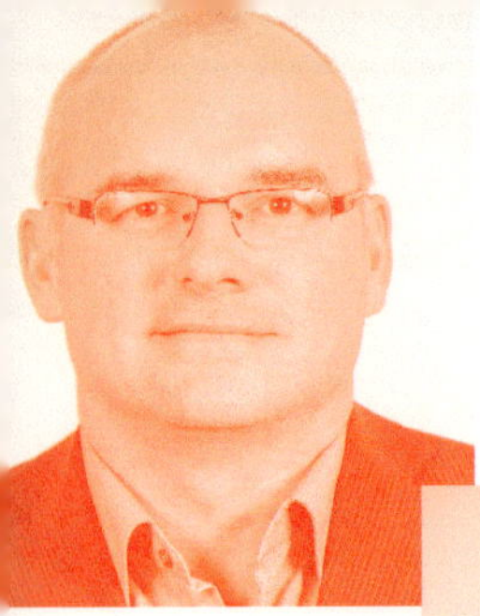
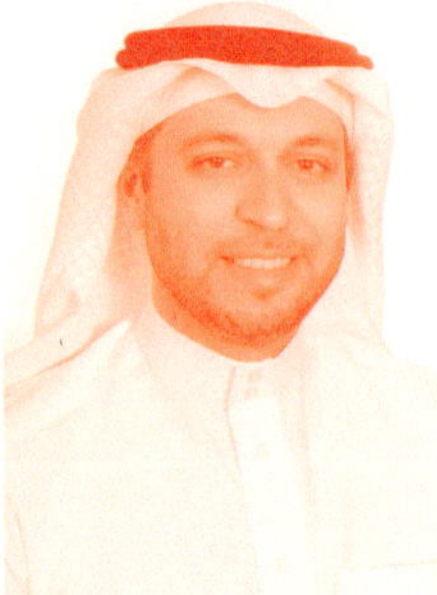
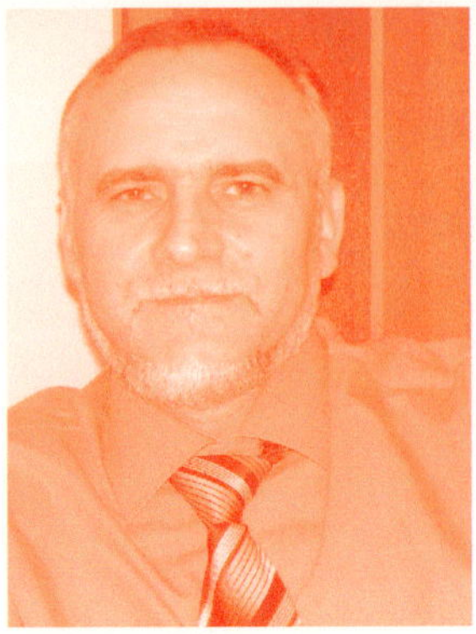
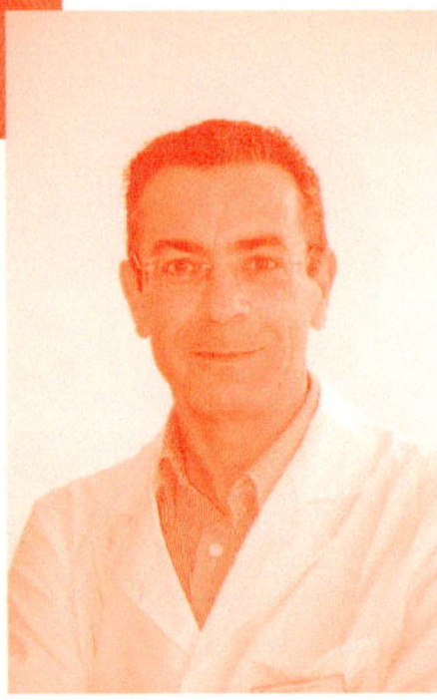
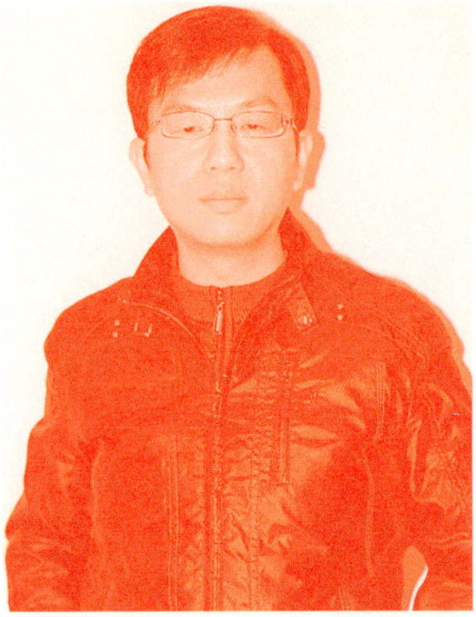
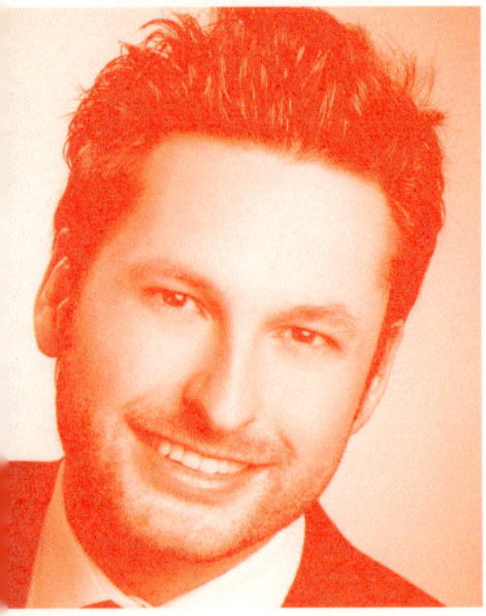
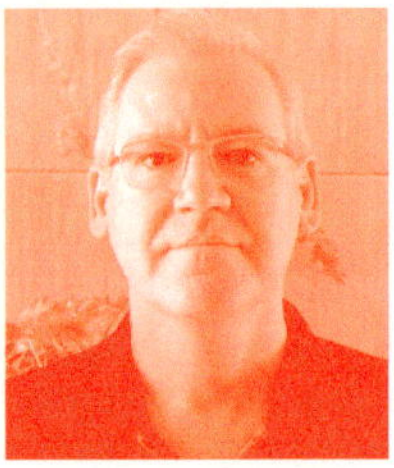

IntechOpen

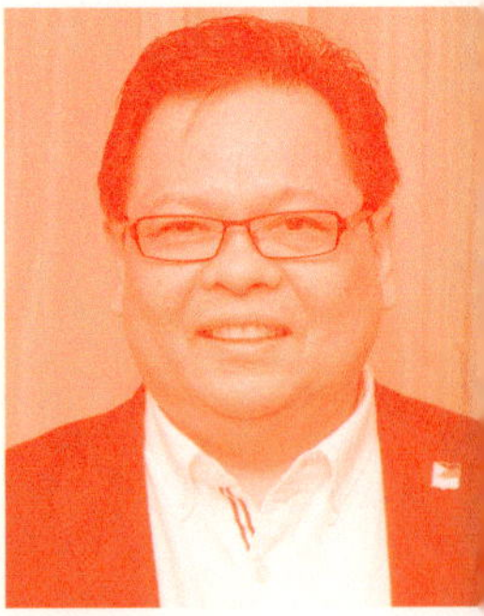
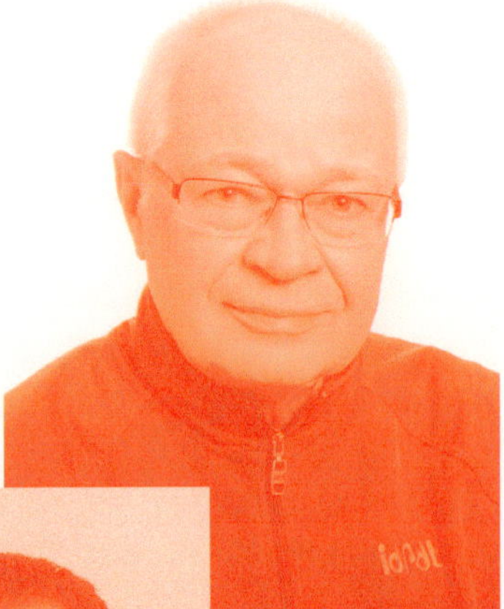
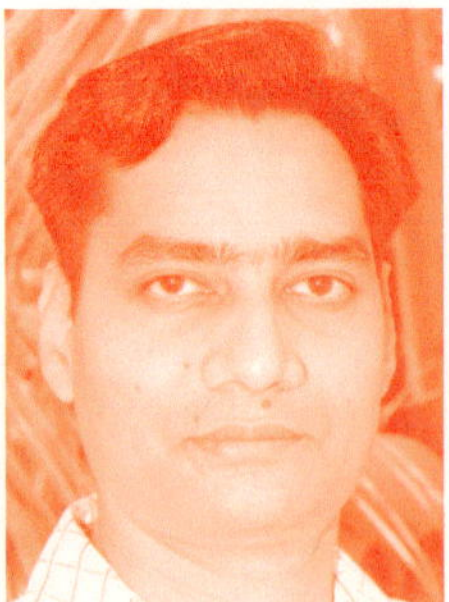
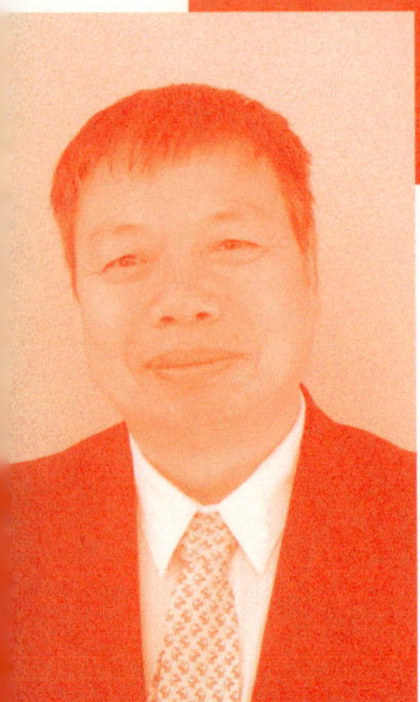
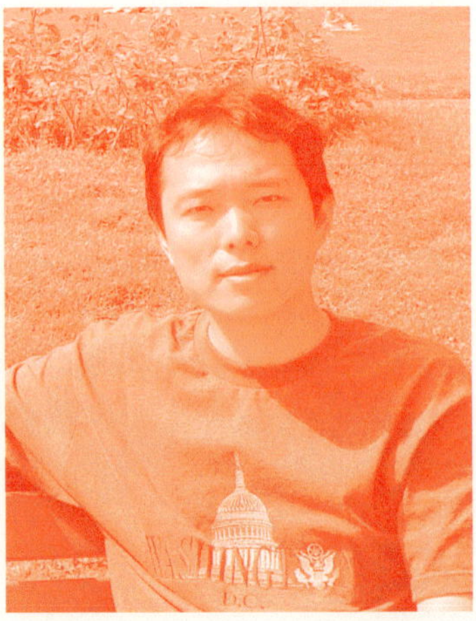
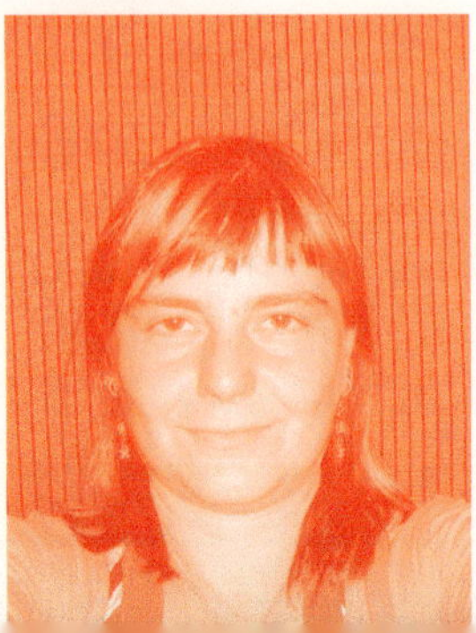

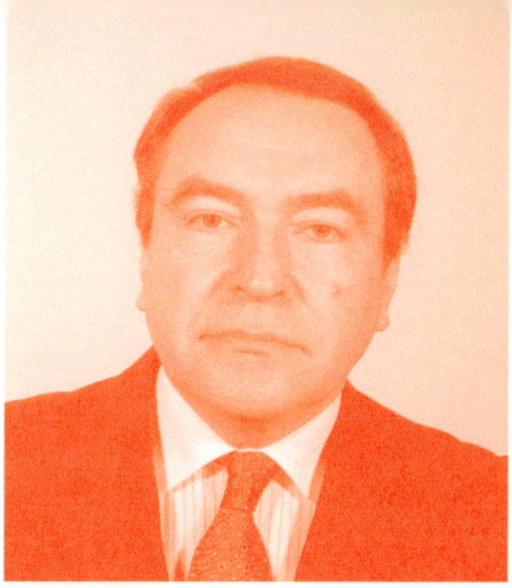
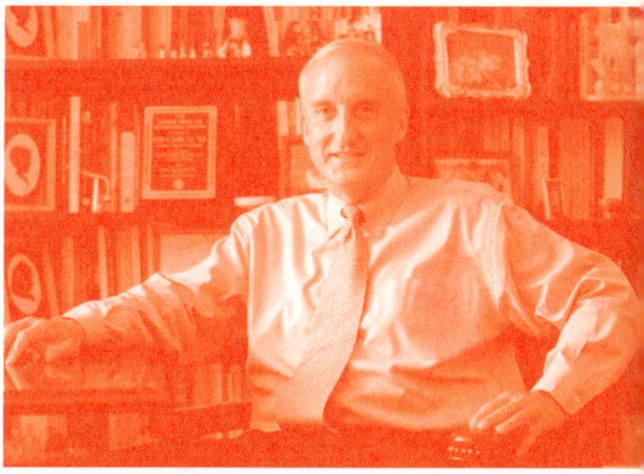
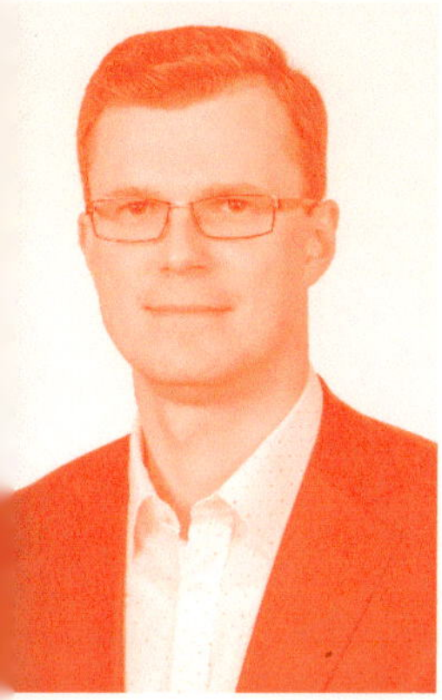
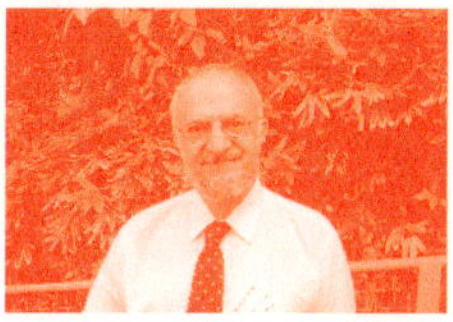
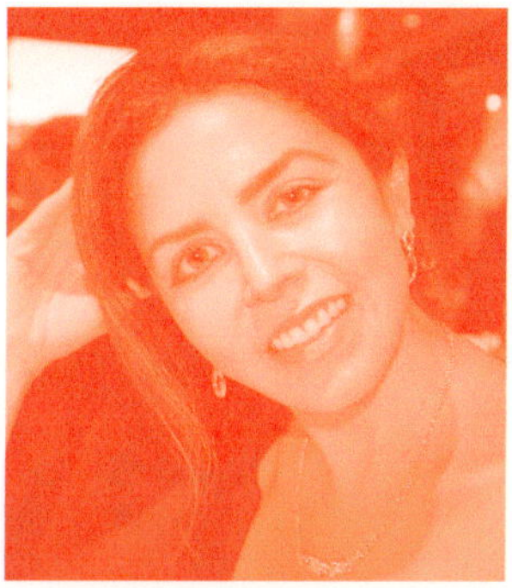

Supporting open minds since 2005

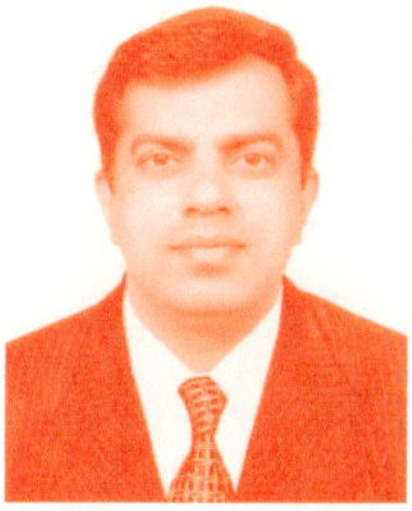
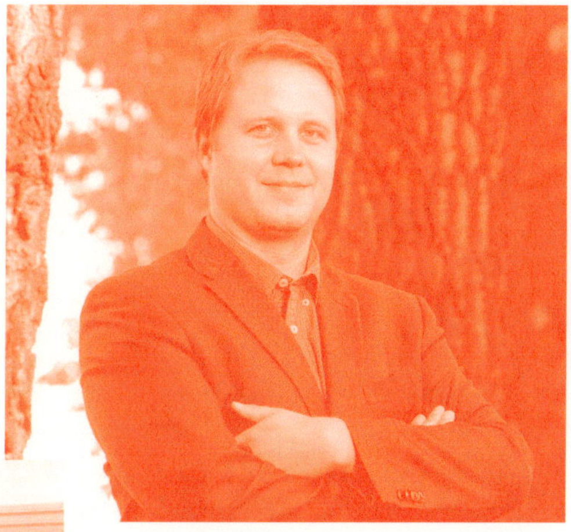
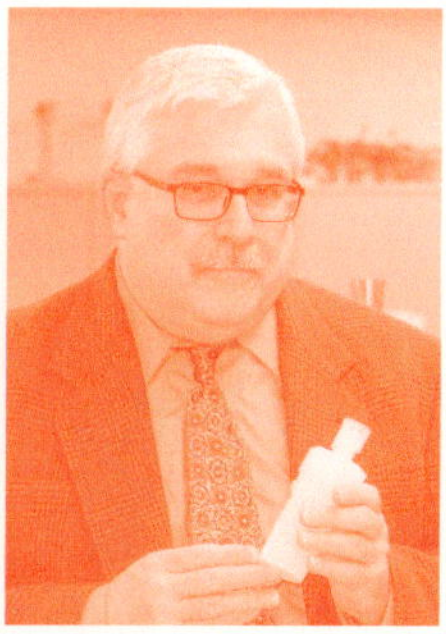
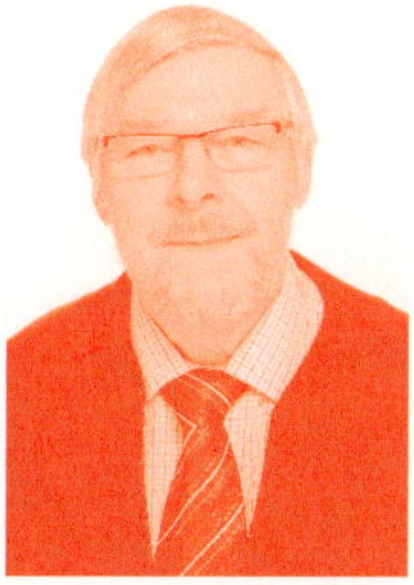
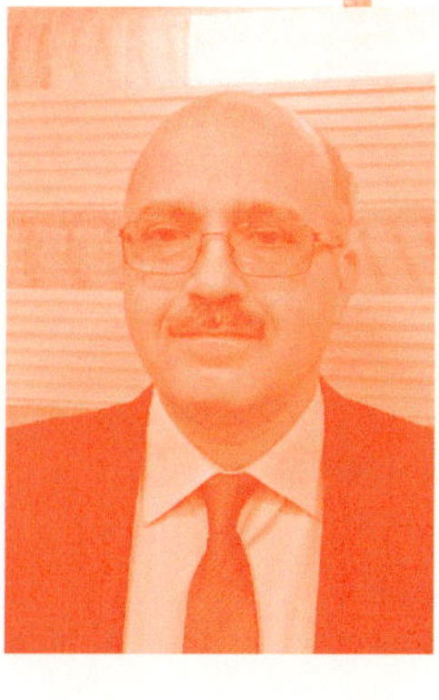
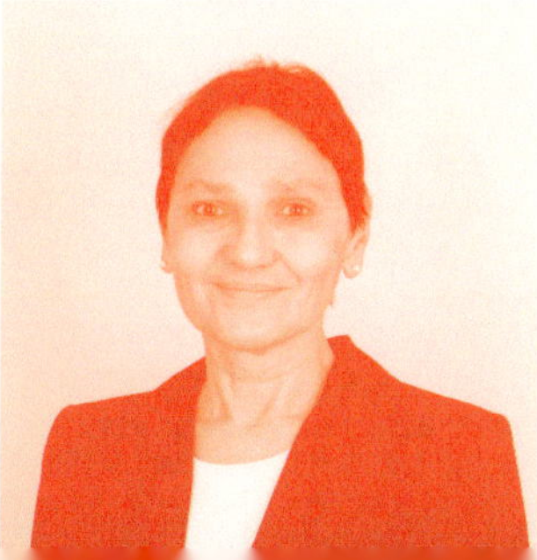
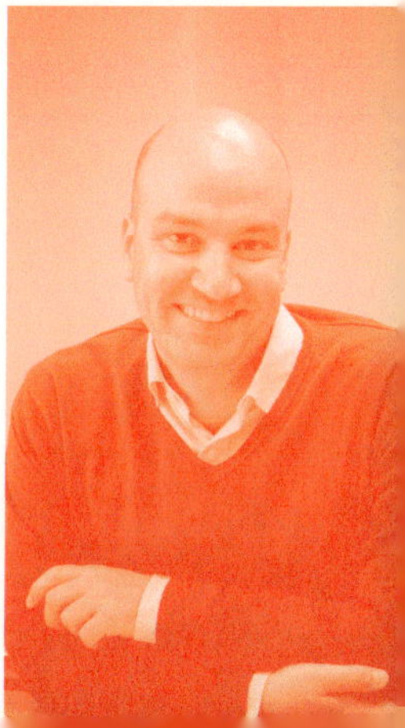

Behavioral Pharmacology - From Basic to Clinical Research
http://dx.doi.org/10.5772/intechopen.77701
Edited by Juan Francisco Rodríguez-Landa and Jonathan Cueto-Escobedo

Contributors
Rosa Isela García-Ríos, Armando Mora- Pérez, Cesar Soria-Fregozo, Ana Raquel Ramos-Molina, Gabriel Guillén-Ruiz, Blandina Bernal-Morales, Emma Virgina Herrera-Huerta, Ana Karen Limón-Vázquez, Margarita Hernández-Mixteco, Abraham Puga-Olguín, Socorro Herrera-Meza, Rafael Fernández-Demeneghi, Isidro Vargas-Moreno, Rosa Isela Guzmán-Gerónimo, Yolanda Campos-Uscanga, Tania Romo-Gonzalez, Héctor-Gabriel Acosta-Mesa, Lorena-Guadalupe Patraca-Camacho, Juan Francisco Rodríguez-Landa, Jonathan Cueto-Escobedo, Fabio García-García, Caio Maximino, Minerva Hernández Lozano, Marcos Fernando Ocaña-Sanchez, Rosa Virginia García Rodríguez, Libna Sulem Gallardo Beatriz, Ibrahim Castro Torres, María Gabriela Alcántara López, Julio César González Ortiz, Tania Monserrat Camacho Márquez, Gabriela Josefina Mendoza Rangel, Van Dan Castro Gerónimo, María Angélica Ocampo Ocampo, Popoca Sanchez César Guillermo, Abraham Sánchez, Catalina Casillas, Raúl Cicero

First published in London, United Kingdom, 2020 by IntechOpen
IntechOpen is the global imprint of INTECHOPEN LIMITED, registered in England and Wales, registration number: 11086078, 5 Princes Gate Court, London, SW7 2QJ, United Kingdom
Printed in Croatia

British Library Cataloguing-in-Publication Data
A catalogue record for this book is available from the British Library

Additional hard and PDF copies can be obtained from orders@intechopen.com

Behavioral Pharmacology - From Basic to Clinical Research
Edited by Juan Francisco Rodríguez-Landa and Jonathan Cueto-Escobedo
p. cm.
Print ISBN 978-1-78985-679-8
Online ISBN 978-1-78985-680-4
eBook (PDF) ISBN 978-1-83880-574-6

For EU product safety concerns:
IN TECH d.o.o., Prolaz Marije Krucifikse Kozulić 3, 51000 Rijeka, Croatia, info@intechopen.com or visit our website at intechopen.com.

Meet the editors

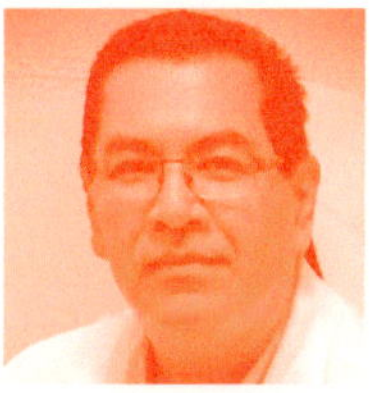

Juan Francisco Rodríguez-Landa received his doctorate degree in Psychology (Behavioral Neuroscience) from the Universidad Nacional Autónoma de México (UNAM). He is a full-time researcher at the Laboratory of Neuropharmacology, Institute of Neuroethology, Universidad Veracruzana. He is a lecturer in Neuropsychopharmacology and belongs to the National System of Investigators (SNI 2) and Mexican Academy of Sciences. His research interests include the effects of neurosteroids and natural products on anxiety, depression, and neuronal activity in some brain structures related to anxiety and depression disorders. He has published multiple specialized scientific papers, book chapters, and books. He is an expert journal peer reviewer and active member of the European Behavioral Pharmacology Society, International Society for Neuroethology, and Mexican Society of Physiological Sciences, among others.

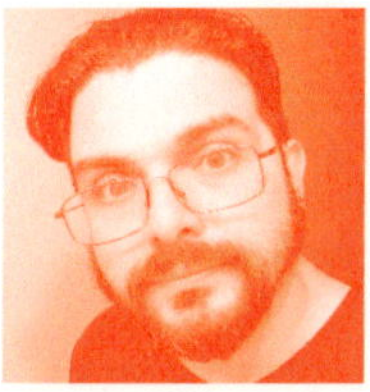

Jonathan Cueto-Escobedo received his doctorate degree in Psychology (Behavioral Neuroscience) from the Universidad Nacional Autónoma de México. He is currently a researcher at the Institute of Health Sciences, Universidad Veracruzana and a member of the National System of Investigators (SNI I). His research interests include experimental models of anxiety and depression, neurobiology of behavior, particularly addiction and food intake as a reward with a translational perspective. He has published 10 book chapters and 13 scientific papers and made more than 20 presentations at international conferences. He has also published several works of science divulgation. He has lectured at several universities in México, including the University of Xalapa, University of Veracruz, University of Guadalajara, University of Tlaxcala, and Universidad Nacional Autónoma de México.

Contents

Preface

Behavioral Pharmacology is a multidisciplinary science of the neurosciences. The principal focus is based on the study of the biological bases of drugs that influence the normal or altered behavior. This science explores the link between physiological and neurobiological processes with those drugs, hormones, and natural compounds impacting on behavior. This science studies the biological effects of drugs through behavioral analysis, which is mostly supported by chemical or physiological correlations that explain the expression of a specific behavior. Research in this area has substantially contributed to the understanding of neurobiology and neuropharmacology of psychiatric disorders, neurodegenerative disorders, as well as eating and sleeping disorders, and addictions to drugs, among others. Nowadays, research into pharmacology has grown beyond treatments for infectious agents, and into areas covering the neurobiological bases of diseases related to alterations of the central nervous system. Derived from those studies, we now dispose of pharmacological therapies to treat several disorders such as depression, anxiety, chronic pain, attention deficit, psychomotor hyperactivity, epilepsy, and Parkinson's disease; but also, further studies are in processes to develop efficacious medicines to ameliorate Alzheimer's disease. One of the most important current health problems is related to the addictive behaviors triggered by the consumption of certain substances and the side effects of these addictions, including the consumption of tobacco, alcohol, and refined sugars, that impact negatively on quality of life. The current technological development has a significant impact on mental health for example the Internet and smartphone addiction. All these highlight the continuous development of behavioral pharmacology in order to cope with the current challenges to prevent the deterioration of mental health. Behavioral Pharmacology has contributed to development of techniques focused on screening the effects of pharmacological agents on specific behaviors under controlled environments; which allows scientists to work with validated models using the analysis of specific behaviors (i.e., exploration, ambulation, rearing or grooming, among others) or a group of them to identify, for example, the sexual behavior (i.e., number of mounts, latency and number of ejaculations, among others). All of these behaviors are normally studied in experimental subjects under controlled environments designed specifically for the required behavioral display, in which the effects of new chemical agents with potential therapeutic applications are evaluated and contrasted with clinical effective drugs. In summary, the development of behavioral pharmacology permits the study of the biological bases of behavior and the pharmacological action of several substances through the behavioral analysis, contributing to the discovery of substances to maintain an adequate quality of life. Taken together, through behavioral pharmacology it is possible to generate knowledge about pharmacological bases that influence the normal or altered behavior with a multidisciplinary point of view that includes diverse areas of science. So, the purpose of this book "Behavioral Pharmacology - From Basic to Clinical Research" is to show the advances in the identification of pharmacological properties of natural and synthetic molecules that could be used in the development of pharmacological therapies to ameliorate symptoms that affect the wellness of the population, but also of several strategies to prevent the use of addictive abuse. Thanks to all the contributing authors, external reviewers, and the Author Service Manager, we hope you find these efforts satisfactory and wish you a good reading.

Juan Francisco Rodríguez-Landa, PhD
Institue of Neuroethology,
Universidad Veracruzana,
México

Jonathan Cueto-Escobedo, PhD
Institue of Health Sciences,
Universidad Veracruzana,
México

Chapter 1

Introductory Chapter: Behavioral Pharmacology - From Basic to Clinical Research

Juan Francisco Rodríguez-Landa and Jonathan Cueto-Escobedo

1. Behavioral pharmacology

Behavioral pharmacology is a multidisciplinary field of science focused on exploring and understanding the effects of chemical substances, hormones, and drugs on the behavior of humans and experimental animals, all with the final objective of understanding the neurobiological substrate of behavior and contributing in the development of therapeutic agents or pharmacologic tools for research in neurosciences [1]. The relative new popularity and accelerated growth of neurosciences have simultaneously led to an exponential growth on the scientific literature on this area that has been produced every day [2–6]. That makes necessary new strategies to be ready in a field that has been constantly actualized; for example, years ago, students with different backgrounds, who are graduates of psychology, medicine, or chemistry, had to study postgraduate trainings to specialize in the field of neurosciences. Nowadays, students from diverse universities can apply a career in "neurosciences" that has been recently designed by the National Autonomous University of Mexico few years ago [7]. This is an example on how universities have adapted to offer a better preparation on neurosciences fields. In this sense, the present book also attempts to offer the reader a source of current knowledge in behavioral pharmacology from different backgrounds.

Despite the relatively brief history of the behavioral pharmacology, it has significantly contributed in the understanding of the importance of the environmental and behavioral factors that determine the effect of drugs and chemical compounds with potential therapeutic and toxicological actions that impact on the health of the human being or another organisms [8]. In this way, the experimental and clinical procedures into the behavioral pharmacology have permitted the identification of natural or synthetic substances with potential utility in the treatment of central nervous system disorders, including anxiety, depression, and Alzheimer's and Parkinson's diseases [9–15], among others.

In support, the present book is a multidisciplinary compilation that illustrates the advancement and development of behavioral pharmacology supported in areas as pharmacology and psychology, experimental analysis of behavior, psychophysiology, and the recently called neurosciences such as neuroethology, neurophysiology, and neurochemistry, among others. In this book, the authors included and discussed results in the field of behavioral pharmacology and neurosciences. The chapters include scientific information derived from basic research in laboratory animals and the impact that this information has in the development of potential pharmacological treatments to be applied in the clinical research to contribute in the wellness of the human being. The relevance of these contributions is the discussion of the experimental analysis of behavior under diverse pharmacological treatments, including complementary results from neurochemistry, neuropharmacology, neurophysiology, psychopharmacology, neuroanatomy, and molecular biology that permit the identification of the mechanism of action involved in the potential beneficial and toxic effects of the evaluated drugs.

2. Author's contribution to the present book

Cueto-Escobedo and collaborators (Chapter 2) show a brief history of the development of behavioral pharmacology over the years, as well as the contribution of this science in the development of animal models that have contributed in the knowledge of the biological bases of behavior and importantly in the identification of potential therapeutic and toxic agents that may impact on the central nervous system disorder. Fernández-Demeneghi and collaborators (Chapter 3) report how identifying the potential beneficial effects of functional food on health has been possible through the use of the techniques of behavioral pharmacology. In this case they report the effects of berry juice or its secondary metabolites (i.e., polyphenols, anthocyanins, and other constituents) on some central nervous system disorders like anxiety, depression, Alzheimer's and Parkinson's diseases, and cognitive alterations. Hernandez-Lozano and collaborators (Chapter 4) discuss the potential use of botanical and natural pharmaceutical resources in the management of neuropathy pain based on preclinical studies. Additionally, include relevant information about of the phytochemical, toxicity, adverse effects, and biosecurity reported to botanical and natural pharmaceutical resources used in pain control.

The evaluation of natural products or new synthetic molecules with potential application in the treatment of symptoms that impact on the wellness of animals or human beings firstly may be based on exploring their effects in a traditional context (i.e., using extracts, infusions, or juice), but derived from these studies, a more specific screening is focused on isolated, characterized, and purified secondary metabolites, where a more controlled dosage may be realized. Garcia-Rios and collaborators (Chapter 5) describe and discuss preclinical results of specific plant secondary metabolites and their potential use in clinical therapy of anxiety and depression, which is compared with clinically effective anxiolytic and antidepressant drugs. Particularly, the anxiolytic and antidepressant effects of terpenes, flavonoids, alkaloids, and sterols and their mechanism of action on the central nervous system are discussed.

Behavioral pharmacology studies also had contributed in understanding neurobehavioral bases that underlie some psychiatric disorders and the pharmacological action of drugs in a specific context. Guillen-Ruiz and collaborators (Chapter 6) provide a general overview of the usefulness of animal behavioral models to explore the anxiety disorders in childhood and its neurobiological bases and to then explore potential anxiolytic therapies to minimizing side effects in this particular population. Finally, Ocampo-Ocampo and collaborators (Chapter 7) address the problem of addiction and their treatment from behavioral analysis and an integrative holistic approach, with the aim of preventing or reducing the physical and mental damage that addictive substances may cause to the health, improving the quality of life of psychoactive substance consumers.

3. Concluding remarks

This short chapter must be considered to be a brief and necessarily incomplete review that has the only purpose of introducing the works of the authors in the next chapters to the reader. As you can see, behavioral pharmacology has brought great progress in the understanding of the neurobiology of different central nervous system disorders and in the understanding of the mechanism of action of drugs used to treat such disorders, as those mentioned in this chapter and the whole book. We hope the present work will enrich your knowledge on the study of behavioral pharmacology.

Author details

Juan Francisco Rodríguez-Landa[1,2]* and Jonathan Cueto-Escobedo[3]

1 Laboratory of Neuropharmacology, Institute of Neuroethology, Universidad Veracruzana, Xalapa, Veracruz, México

2 Faculty of Biological Pharmaceutical Chemistry, Universidad Veracruzana, Xalapa, Veracruz, México

3 Translational and Clinical Research Department, Institute of Health Sciences, Universidad Veracruzana, Xalapa, Veracruz, México

*Address all correspondence to: juarodriguez@uv.mx

References

[1] Branch MN. Behavioral pharmacology. In: Lattal EA, Iversen IH, editors. Experimental Analysis of Behavior. Amsterdam: Elsevier; 1991. pp. 21-70

[2] Branch MN. How research in behavioral pharmacology informs behavioral science. Journal of the Experimental Analysis of Behavior. 2006;**85**(3):407-423. DOI: 10.1901/jeab.2006.130-04

[3] Planchez B, Surget A, Belzung C. Animal models of major depression: Drawbacks and challenges. Journal of Neural Transmission. 2019;**126**(11):1383-1408. DOI: 10.1016/j.neurol.2015.07.011

[4] Kuhn BN, Kalivas PW, Bobadilla AC. Understanding addiction using animal models. Frontiers in Behavioral Neuroscience. 2019;**13**:262. DOI: 10.3389/fnbeh.2019.00262

[5] Maximino C, Arndt SS, van der Staay FJ. Animal models. In: Vonk J, Schackelford TK, editors. Encyclopedia of Animal Cognition and Behavior. Basel: Springer Nature Switzerland; 2019. pp. 1-17

[6] Ferreira GS, Veening-Griffioen D, Boon W, Moors E, de Gispen-de Wied C, Schellekens H, et al. A standardized framework to identify optimal animal models for efficacy assessment in drug development. PLOS One. 2019;**14**(6):e0218014

[7] Nacional Autonomous University of Mexico (UNAM), Faculty of Medicine, Bachelor degree in Neurosciences. Mexico City: Neurosciences UNAM. 2020. Available from: http://neurociencias.facmed.unam.mx [Accessed: 03 March 2020]

[8] Chast F. A History of Drug Discovery: From First Steps of Chemistry to Achievements in Molecular Pharmacology. London: Academic Press; 2008. pp. 3-62

[9] Bourin M. Experimental anxiety model for anxiety disorders: Relevance to drug discovery. In: Kim YK, editor. Anxiety Disorders. Advances in Experimental Medicine and Biology. Singapore: Springer; 2020. pp. 169-184

[10] Robbins TW, Murphy ER. Behavioural pharmacology: 40+ years of progress, with a focus on glutamate receptors and cognition. Trends in Pharmacological Sciences. 2006;**27**(3):141-148. DOI: 10.1016/j.tips.2006.01.009

[11] Marr MJ. Behavioral pharmacology: Issues of reductionism and causality. In: Barrett JE, Thompson T, Dews P, editors. Advances in Behavioral Pharmacology. Hillsdale: Lawrence Erlbaum; Vol. 7. 1990. p. 1-12

[12] Rodríguez-Landa JF, Hernández-Figueroa JD, Hernández-Calderón BC, Saavedra M. Anxiolytic-like effect of phytoestrogen genistein in rats with long-term absence of ovarian hormones in the black and white model. Progress in Neuropsychopharmacology and Biological Psychiatry. 2009;**33**(2):367-372. DOI: 10.1016/j.pnpbp.2008.12.024

[13] Rodríguez-Landa JF, Puga-Olguín A, Germán-Ponciano LJ, Olmos-Vázquez OJ, Bernal-Morales B. Phytoestrogens as potential therapeutic agents for the treatment of anxiety and affective disorders. In: Atta-ur-Rahman, editor. Studies in Natural Products Chemistry. Vol. 58. Amsterdam: Elsevier; 2018. pp. 133-159

[14] Rodríguez-Landa JF, Hernández-López F, Cueto-Escobedo J, Herrera-Huerta EV, Rivadeneyra-Domínguez E,

Bernal-Morales B, et al. Chrysin (5,7-dihydroxyflavone) exerts anxiolytic-like effects through GABAA receptors in a surgical menopause model in rats. Biomedicine & Pharmacotherapy. 2019;**109**:2387-2395. DOI: 10.1016/j.biopha.2018.11.111

[15] Rodríguez-Landa JF, Olmos-Vázquez OJ, Dutra-da-Costa BP, Lima-Maximino M, Maximino C, Guillén-Ruiz G. Action of progesterone on depression-like behavior in a model of surgical menopause are mediated by GABAA receptors. Salud Mental. 2020;**43**(1):43-53. DOI: 10.17711/SM.0185-3325.2020.007

Chapter 2

New Developments in Behavioral Pharmacology

Jonathan Cueto-Escobedo, Fabio García-García, Caio Maximino and Juan Francisco Rodríguez-Landa

Abstract

Behavioral pharmacology research has been a cornerstone in the understanding of the processes that underlie the behavior of living organisms as well as the biological basis of the behavioral, emotional, and cognitive disorders that affect humans. The findings in this area have helped to explore the potential therapeutic effects of several substances for the treatment of the mentioned disorders. The present chapter brings an extremely brief introduction to this vast area. First, we try to put in context behavioral pharmacology and its relevance and then show some brief examples of how this discipline has developed over the years. Second, we review the concept of a "research model" in preclinical behavioral pharmacology, given the importance of animal models and tests in this area, followed by a brief review of the recent advances using zebra fish as a valuable tool of research. Third, more specific examples are aborded, such as the findings on sleep disorders and those related to sexual hormones and menopause.

Keywords: behavioral pharmacology, psychopharmacology, psychoactive drugs, behavioral models

1. Introduction

Every time academics talk about the evolution of human societies and the advance of humanity, language is always mentioned, followed by different pieces of technology that allowed us to change the world. Few times, medicine is mentioned, and within the same area of knowledge, pharmacology is even more frequently omitted. But without the development of pharmacology as a science founded in systematic research, the capacities of medical sciences and therapeutics would be very limited. Knowledge in pharmacology allows us to understand that there exist chemical substances with very specific structures and properties which, in controlled doses, can interact with the normal physiology of our organism in order to produce effects that improve our health, known as therapeutic effects; but if the doses are insufficient or excessive, the effects will be useless or harmful (toxic), respectively [1]. These substances responsible for the actions of medicines are named as active compounds.

Most of the active compounds used in medicine were consumed together with the organism which contained them, most frequently plants. As chemistry advanced, scientists succeed in isolating these compounds and described their chemical structure. In consequence, laboratories started to synthesize these substances and others with a similar structure that should be tested in research laboratories before using them to treat diseases in humans [2].

Nowadays, pharmacological research has grown beyond treatments for infectious agents, covering diseases related to the alteration of the normal functioning of the central nervous system (CNS). There are medications to treat disorders such as depression, anxiety, chronic pain, attention deficit and hyperactivity disorder, epilepsy, and Parkinson's disease, and new drugs are desperately sought to stop Alzheimer's disease. On the other hand, one of the most important current health problems is related to the addictive behaviors triggered by the consumption of certain substances and the side effects of these addictions: respiratory and cardiovascular diseases in the case of tobacco, metabolic diseases in the case of alcoholism and addictive consumption of refined sugars, infectious diseases in the case of injected drugs, and many others that are not mentioned here. Without losing sight of the fact that addiction is itself a disease of the nervous system with devastating effects *per se* on the patient's quality of life. In several countries, prescription of different therapeutic agents acting on the CNS to treat psychiatric disorders, such as antidepressants, antipsychotics, and stimulants, has increased [3, 4] as in the case of methylphenidate and amphetamines in different countries such as United States [5] and the Netherlands [6]. The same way, antidepressant users have increased markedly around the world in countries such as Norway, Sweden, and Denmark [7], among others. Additionally, the use of different substances of abuse such as tobacco [8] and marijuana has increased in the population [9]. Also, the development of new technologies and products has a significant impact on mental health as the discovery of Internet addiction [10] and the addictive consumption of refining sugar [11, 12], which impacts on the behavior of subjects. All these make important the continuous development of behavioral pharmacology in order to cope with the challenges in mental health.

2. Development of behavioral pharmacology

Behavioral pharmacology, also known as psychopharmacology, has developed as an interdisciplinary science that comprises fields such as neuroethology, neurochemistry, pharmacology and neuropharmacology, psychophysiology, neurophysiology, experimental analysis of behavior, and several other fields related to neurosciences [13]. Behavioral pharmacology is founded on systematic research with precise methods for assessing and interpreting the effects of chemical, hormones, and drugs on the behavior in humans and experimental animals in order to establish its potential as therapeutic agents or pharmacologic tools to explore how the brain functions and the underlying neurobiological mechanism of cognition, emotions, and behavior. Behavioral pharmacology must thus be an integral component of many neuroscience research programs [14].

In this sense, the development of behavioral pharmacology comprises the development of areas as pharmacology and psychology, experimental analysis of behavior, and recently neuroscience. For a historical review, see [14–16]. However, research in behavioral pharmacology can be summarized in: (1) the development of procedures to screen pharmacological agents for potential clinical effectiveness. (2) Perfecting behavioral techniques to explore the mechanisms of action of behaviorally active drugs and using these chemicals and drugs as tools for the analysis of complex behaviors (i.e., when drugs reinforce behavior and when drugs serve as discriminative stimuli) [16] (see **Table 1**). Therefore, drugs are not only a subject of study, because of its behavioral effects but are also a piece of technology that helps to elucidate how behaviors are controlled by living organisms.

Year	Description	Reference
1936	Selye H. described the impact of several types of adverse stimuli on animal health, in the form of a syndrome characterized by three phases: alarm, adaptation, and exhaustion, which can lead to death if stimuli are maintained. This syndrome was later named as the stress response which has been intensively studied and strongly associated with the impairment of brain function in animals or the development of mental disorders in humans	[17]
1972	The first study to administrate Delta-9-tetrahydrocannabinol in humans to test the effects on sleep patterns is carried out. The results show a decrease in sleep onset latency. To date, there are controversial results about the positive effects the cannabis on sleep quality	[18]
1977	The forced swim test is proposed as a behavioral tool to explore the effects of antidepressant drugs in rats and mice that are exposed to a stressful inescapable condition that triggers despair behavior (immobility)	[19]
1986	Elevated plus maze is developed as a tool to measure anxiety-like behaviors of the rat and test substances with potential anxiolytic effects	[20]
1988	Modafinil was prescribed for the first time for the treatment of narcolepsy and idiopathic hypersomnia in patients	[21]
2005	This study explored the behavioral and neuronal response to stress in ovariectomized rats (OVX). These rats were more sensitive to stress, which was associated with a low concentration of steroid hormones. This effect was prevented by restitution with 17-β estradiol	[22]
2006	Anxiety-like behavior is dependent on the post-ovariectomy time frame. At 12-week post-ovariectomy there is more anxiety-like behavior than a 3-week post-ovariectomy	[23]
2016	The first systemic review and meta-analysis that discuss the effects of the orexin agonist Suvorexant for the treatment of insomnia. Suvorexant improved some sleep parameters, but some adverse effects were reported	[24]
2019	In this study, it was identified that at 3-week post-ovariectomy appears anxiety-like behavior, but from 6-week post-ovariectomy in addition to anxiety-like behavior, also increases depression-like behavior in rats, supporting an experimental model of surgical post-menopause	[25]

Table 1.
Emblematic research in behavioral pharmacology.

3. Measuring behavior

Behavior is a biological property of organisms, which remarks on the significance of the study of drug-behavior interactions [15]. Maybe, a great example of the impact of behavior beyond psychology is the research by ethologists K. Lorenz, N. Tinbergen, and K. von Frisch, which focused on the analysis of behavior in several species including fish, insects, and birds, and the importance of which made them worthy of the Nobel price of medicine in 1973 "*for their discoveries concerning organization and elicitation of individual and social behaviour patterns*."

The first step in all behavioral sciences has been to define what is behavior; it could seem an easy task, but historically many different definitions of behavior have been used by scientists over the time, and even the knowing of a unique definition is elusive and may be useless for every different area such as psychology, ethology, and experimental analysis of behavior, among others; for review see [26, 27]. As mentioned before, one of the directions of behavioral pharmacology was the development of procedures to screen the effects of pharmacological agents on specific behaviors under controlled environments. This approach allows scientists to work with operational definitions of specific behaviors, for example, exploration can be measured by scoring ambulation, rearing or nose approaching to an object; sexual behavior can be measured by conditioned place preference, number of mounts, latency and number of ejaculations. All these behaviors are normally studied under controlled environments that are designed specifically to the required behavioral display and every feature of the environment; the experimental subjects or chemical agents with probed effects on humans have been studied in this environment with the purpose of establishing these manipulations as models of a specific behavior (see **Table 2**) as spatial learning and memory, or models of specific pathologies behaviorally expressed as is the case of anxiety [28], depression [29], obsessive compulsive disorder [30], Parkinson [31], epilepsy [32] or addictive behaviors [33], and sleep deprivation [34], among others.

3.1 Behavioral models of brain disorders

Animals are used as proxies for human phenomena throughout the literature, and the exact definition of what constitutes a "model" can be confusing. In behavioral pharmacology, a field that intersects between psychology, neuroscience, and pharmacology [42], different uses are attributed to different epistemic operations and, as a consequence, to different definitions of validity [43, 44]. One of the most basic definitions is that by Paul Willner, which defined screening tests as those uses of animal behavior that are capable of discriminating between different drug effects (i.e., possess high predictive validity); behavioral bioassays as those uses of animal behavior that are capable of shedding light on the neural basis of normal behavior (i.e., possess high

Research area	Description
Hormone restitution therapy	This review discussed, 25 years ago, the importance of steroid hormones in the regulation of behavior and some psychiatry disorders; particularly depression associated with premenstrual syndrome and the transition to menopause. Also, it discusses some research about the role of hormone restitution therapy in ameliorating depression symptoms [35]
Sexual dimorphism	This review discusses preclinical and clinical research that show how hormones are involved in the sex differences in some psychiatric disorders like anxiety, and their interactions between fear, stress, and gonadal hormones [36]
Behavioral animal models	This research reviews the relevance of non-mammalian models in behavioral pharmacology with application in the development of biological psychiatry [37]
Behavioral model of menopause	This review highlights the importance of animal models of menopause in the understanding of neurobiological changes associated with the long-term absence of ovarian hormones. To then elucidate novel perspectives and interventions to improve the life quality in the menopausal women under a translational context [38]
Sleep and insomnia	This review describes the efficacy of new drugs in the treatment of insomnia such as melatonin, Remelteon, Tasimelteon, and Suvorexant, among others [39]
Hormones and behavior	This review discusses the influence of hormones on brain function and behavior, and integrate information to explain how the brain and the body communicate reciprocally via hormones and other mediators, and in ways that influence brain and body health but which can also accelerate diseases processes when the mediators of allostasis are dysregulated [40]
Addiction	A review of the most popular behavioral models for the study of addictions such as conditioned place preference and self-administration and new models to study behavioral addictions as gambling and exercise addiction [33]
Sleep disorders	This review describes the Pitolisant (Wakix®), first-in-class antagonist/inverse agonist of the H3 receptor for the treatment of narcolepsy with or without cataplexy [41]

Table 2.
Current topics in behavioral pharmacology.

face validity); and simulations as those uses of animal behavior that can inform on the etiology, pathophysiology, and treatment of human (mental) disorders (i.e., possess high construct validity). Further developments of this framework [45] advance the theory of validity, therefore improving the capability of researchers to evaluate animal models.

Screening tests show good predictive validity in that they are able to detect the effects of drugs, which are already known to have clinical efficacy; as a result, they are likely to be able to predict the effect of new drugs, which show similar biochemical or behavioral effects in the test [42, 43]. Examples include most uses of the tail suspension test and forced swim tests, which are commonly referred to as models of depression but actually do not simulate the etiological and pathophysiological aspects of human depression. When used without any further manipulations of the animal (i.e., lesions, genetic manipulations, or other stressors which are thought to be causally related to depression), these tests are good at discriminating drugs which act as serotonin reuptake inhibitors and reasonably good at predicting antidepressant efficacy. Since screening tests rely mostly on predictive validity, current approaches to modeling in behavioral pharmacology view them as limited. Moreover, producing models which show good construct validity in at least some domains (i.e., epidemiology, symptomatology and natural history, genetics, biochemistry, etiology, histological alterations, or endpoints) has been proposed as a way to indirectly increase predictive validity [46], as drugs which improve performance in a test that simulates at least some aspects of the target disorder.

Behavioral bioassays are tests that use nonhuman animals to try to understand the histological, electrophysiological, biochemical, and genetic bases of neurobehavioral functions [42, 43]. Usually, bioassays are used to understand normal functioning, instead of pathological alterations in these psychological processes. They rely on face validity—that is, how much performance in the test "resembles" the target human function. Of course, taken "as is," face validity runs a great risk of anthropomorphism, and the resemblance should not be sought at the topography level, but at the functional level [47]. For example, the elevated plus-maze, when used as a test *per se* (and not as an endpoint in a simulation), is interpreted as a behavioral bioassay of anxiety due to the functional role of thigmotaxis in rodent defensive behavior [48, 49]. Of course, this comparison only makes sense if we consider that anxiety is a normal mechanism that is associated with defensive behavior [50, 51]. Thus, the face validity of a test is only as good as our psychological/behavioral theory about a given function (i.e., anxiety, fear, memory, and attention, among others) [47].

Finally, simulations are tests, which use nonhuman animals to try to understand a human disorder from the point of view of etiology and pathophysiology [42, 43]. Most approaches to psychopathology currently frame disorders in a diathesis-stress theory [45], which assumes that vulnerabilities (general or specific; genetic, developmental, or temperamental) increase the probability of developing a specific disorder when the individual passes through general or specific stressors. In analogy, to develop a simulation of a mental disorder in a nonhuman animal, the vulnerabilities and stressors should be modeled, transforming an "initial organism" into a "vulnerable organism" and this latter into a "pathological organism," in which behavioral endpoints are assessed and biomarkers evaluated [44, 45]. From all senses of "behavioral model," the simulation is the one that better approaches the idea of modeling a disease [42, 44], but is also the more time-consuming. Moreover, to increase the construct validity of a simulation, aspects such as etiology and pathophysiology should be taken into consideration, but sometimes these aspects are unknown and are precisely what is under investigation [42]. Thus, high construct validity needs to be balanced against practical constraints, and therefore no behavioral simulations with optimal characteristics exist [52]. In the next pages some examples of these "behavioral models" are described in order to introduce the present book.

4. Behavioral models in zebra fish

Under the framework discussed above for behavioral models, interesting approaches have appeared using non-rodent species. While mice and rats are still the most widely used model organisms in behavioral pharmacology [53], zebra fish (*Danio rerio* Hamilton 1822) come in an honorable third place, quickly "swimming into view" as a relevant model organism in this field [54]. The "classical" criteria for selecting a model organism in genetics and developmental biology—small size, fast (and external) development, easy reproduction, low cost, genetic tractability [55]—are present in zebra fish [37]. Moreover, other advantages are also described by zebra fish researchers: phylogenetic position; intermediate complexity in physiology and throughput; availability of tools to study neurocircuitry and to interfere in normal function (i.e., expression vectors, pharmacogenomic tools, and advanced microscopy); a productive community of researchers; and accumulation of significant data and methodological developments [37]. The combination of these characteristics suggested that zebra fish could be a suitable model organism in behavioral pharmacology.

Currently, very few true simulations exist in zebra fish, and most behavioral tests that are used to study psychiatric disorders in this species are actually screening tests or behavioral bioassays. This is a consequence of an extensive focus of the research in the field in the last 20 years on developing behavioral tests. This step, of course, was necessary to galvanize research in the field. Notable exceptions exist, but—as is the case with most initial work on using model organisms to study disorders and investigational treatments—these are still limited. However, past research has identified and allowed to control factors that affect zebra fish behavioral tests. Now it is clear how chemical properties of the water, illumination, number of fish per tank and routes of administration modify pharmacological effects. For example, administration by immersion is useful for chronic treatments but lacks a precise control of the doses absorbed [56], on the other hand, intraperitoneal administrations ensure the absolute control of doses but are not useful for chronic treatments due to the stress that produce [57]. Oral administration through drugs incorporated in the food is useful for chronic treatments and controlling the doses is easier than immersion [58], however chemical properties of the drug determine their ability to hold into the food until swallowed and oral metabolism must be considered. With the standardization of the proper protocols these factors can be controlled, and its effects limited so, behavioral pharmacology research with zebra fish is still a suitable and growing field.

The zebra fish light/dark test [59] and the novel tank test [60] are widely used to test the effects of different drugs on anxiety-like behavior in this species. These tests rely on natural preferences observed in the wild, and display excellent remission validity—that is, they are sensitive to drugs which affect anxiety in clinical settings, and not sensitive to drugs which do not affect anxiety [61]. As a result, these tests were used as screening tests to investigate new drugs, including drugs derived from natural products and plants, for example, refs. [62, 63]. These tests have also been used to study the neural mechanisms of anxiety-like behavior [64–68]. Thus, these tests can be used both as screening tests and as behavioral bioassays.

The behavior of adult zebra fish is more complex than the behavior of larvae, but its throughput is smaller. Throughput can be increased by testing larval behavior in microplates [69]. Light levels and stimuli can be delivered simultaneously to many larvae at once, increasing throughput and reproducibility. For example, the photo-motor response (a stereotypic series of motor behaviors that are elicited by high-intensity light) is sensitive to a wide range of psychoactive drugs and able to predict mechanisms of action of drugs, which were previously not investigated in rodents [70]. A battery of assays has been proposed in larval zebra fish that is highly sensitive to antipsychotics and able to identify haloperidol-like compounds [71]. While suffering from the low face and construct validity these assays show very good predictive validity, and therefore are suitable as screening tests.

Examples of simulations can be found in the field of neurological disorders [72]. An interesting example is the generation of mutants with differences in genes known to be associated with diseases. In humans, mutations in the SCN1A gene, which encodes a voltage-gated sodium channel, causes Dravet syndrome, characterized by severe intellectual disability, impaired social development, and drug-resistant seizures. The scn1Lab mutant zebra fish displays spontaneous seizure-like electroencephalogram activity, convulsive-like motor patterns, and hyperactivity [73]. These mutants have been used to investigate drugs, which could be used to treat Dravet syndrome in human patients; drugs that affect the serotonergic system have been found to ameliorate the symptoms in the mutants [74], and suggest interesting avenues for human patients.

Now, we will review the role of behavioral pharmacology on a subject extensively explored in human trials: sleep.

5. Behavioral pharmacology and sleep disorders

Pharmacological treatment of sleep disorders is still partially known and not well understood. Currently, extensively pharmacological research is focused in two sleep disorders: insomnia and narcolepsy. Insomnia is defined as the individual's inability to fall asleep, manifested by a long latency to sleep onset and frequent nighttime awakenings experienced three times per week or more, for at least 1 month [75]. Insomnia causes emotional disturbances, impairs cognition, and reduced quality of life [76, 77]. Most epidemiologic studies have found that about one-third of adults (30–36%) report at least one symptom of insomnia, like difficulty initiating sleep or maintaining sleep [78]. Currently, benzodiazepines or Z-drugs (zopiclone, zolpidem, or zaleplon) are the first options to treat insomnia. These drugs act as positive allosteric modulators at the $GABA_A$ binding site, potentiating GABAergic inhibitory effects [79]. However, short-term or long-term treatment with these drugs has undesirable effects such as cognitive or memory impairment, the rapid development of tolerance, rebound insomnia upon discontinuation, car accidents or falls, and a substantial risk of abuse and dependence [39, 80, 81], which make necessary research on new potential therapeutic agents.

According to the new evidence-based clinical practice guidelines for the treatment of insomnia [75], new pharmacology agents for insomnia management are implemented (**Table 3**).

On the other hand, Type 1 narcolepsy (narcolepsy with hypocretin deficiency) is a chronic neurodegenerative sleep disorder caused by a deficiency of hypocretin-producing neurons in the lateral hypothalamus (LH). Hypocretin neurons are involved in the control of the sleep-wake cycle [87]. Treatment of narcolepsy is traditionally based on amphetamine-like stimulants that enhance dopaminergic release to improve narcoleptic symptoms. Nonetheless, a new group of drugs is arising as a forthcoming treatment of narcolepsy.

Pitolisant (Wakix®) is an inverse agonist of the histamine H3 auto-receptor that not only blocks the braking effect of histamine or H3 receptor agonists on

Drugs	Site of action	Therapeutic effect
Antidepressant (trazodone, mirtazapine, olanzapine, and quetiapine)	Agonists of the serotonin receptor 5-HT_{2A} and 5-HT_{2C}	Moderate improvement in subjective sleep Little improvement in sleep efficiency [82]
Antiparkinsonian ropinirole	Agonist of the dopamine receptor D2	Improvement in efficiency of sleep and total time slept [83]
Suvorexant	Antagonist of the orexin receptor	Improvement of sleep onset and subjective total slept time compared to placebo [84]
Ramelteon	Dual agonist of both MT1 and MT2 melatonin receptors	Improvement in latency to persistent sleep, total sleep time and sleep efficiency [85]
Diphenhydramine	Agonist of the histaminergic receptors	No clear beneficial impact on sleep [86]

Table 3.
New drugs used to insomnia management.

endogenous histamine release from depolarized synaptosomes but also enhances histamine release over the basal level (even at low nanomolar concentrations) in the structures as hypothalamus and cerebral cortex [88]. The administration of 20 mg/kg of Pitolisant promoted wakefulness, and decreased abnormal direct REM sleep onset in narcoleptic hypocretin knockout mice by enhancing histaminergic and noradrenergic activity [89]. Pitolisant seem a safe therapeutic option since doses of 120 mg once a day in the morning, that represent six times the therapeutic, doses did not produce adverse effects and plasma levels reduced at the end of the day, ensuring a lack of waking effect during the night [90]. Additionally, adverse effects due to metabolic drug-drug interaction are low since Pitolisant is metabolized by two distinct CYP_{450} isoforms. For example, the administration of 40 mg of Pitolisant together with 10 mg of Olanzapine to a group of healthy volunteers did not change drug plasma levels compared to only one drug administration [91].

6. Behavioral pharmacology of steroid hormones in a model of surgical menopause

Any chapter on behavioral pharmacology would be incomplete without a section reviewing the effects of certain hormones. Behavioral, emotional and affective states are influenced by plasma and brain concentration of steroid hormones in diverse organisms. Particularly, in nonhuman primates and humans there is significant sexual dimorphism respect to behavior and emotional states. Initially, the attributed properties of steroid hormones were related to the maintaining of secondary sexual characters and reproductive function, but some decades ago, it has been established that steroid hormones also influence behavior and some psychiatric disorders. Expression of anxiety- and depression-related behaviors depends on plasma and brain levels of steroid hormones; which in vulnerable subjects could predispose to development of some psychiatric disorder [92].

In humans, anxiety and depression symptoms are more frequent in women than men in a proportion of 3:1. These differences have been attributed to differences in the concentration of steroid hormones. Particularly in women, a high incidence of anxiety and depression symptoms has been identified during physiological states characterized by low concentration of steroid hormones (i.e., estradiol, progesterone and their reduced metabolites) as naturally occur during premenstrual period, post-partum period, and transition to menopause [93, 94]. However, it also occurs when women are subjected to a surgical procedure to remove the ovaries (i.e., oophorectomy) with or without the uterus (i.e., hysterectomy), where an abrupt reduction in steroid hormones concentrations occurs [95] affecting behavioral response. Apparently, the significant reduction of steroid concentration produces anatomical, physiological, and neurochemical changes in the brain, that negatively impact on behavior, emotional, and affective states [96, 97].

Preclinical research with laboratory animals has made possible identify the behavioral and emotional changes associated with a reduced concentration of steroid hormones when rats are undergoing to an extirpation of both ovaries (i.e., ovariectomy), which increases vulnerability to stress that can be reverted by injection of severe doses of estradiol [22]. The long-term ovariectomy (> 8 weeks post-ovariectomy) is considered then as a surgical menopause model that explores the behavioral, neurobiological, emotional and affective changes associated with oophorectomy that occurs in women [98]. In the long-term ovariectomized rats display higher anxiety- and depression-like behavior in experimental models such as elevated plus maze and forced swim test, respectively. These behavioral changes are correlated with a reduced neurochemical activity on serotonergic, noradrenergic, dopaminergic, and GABAergic pathways; in addition to a reduction in the number of dendritic spines and neuronal activity in some brain structures (i.e., hippocampus, amygdala, lateral septum, prefrontal cortex, among others). Through behavioral analysis is possible identifying the gradual changes associated with surgical menopause in rats. It was observed that after 3-week post-ovariectomy, rats showed high anxiety-like behavior (i.e., there is a reduction of exploration of the open arms) in the elevated plus maze with respect to cycling rats with intact ovaries, but after 6-week post-ovariectomy, additionally to anxiety-like behavior, rats also displayed high depression-like behavior in the forced swim test (i.e., increase in the total time of immobility), which negatively correlates with the Fos-immunoreactive cells in limbic brain structures such as the lateral septal nucleus [25]. The behavioral and neurochemical characterization of long-term ovariectomy allows the pharmacological research of different substances that could be potentially relevant to the development of pharmacological therapies to ameliorate anxiety and depression symptoms that occur during natural or surgical menopause.

As mentioned before, anxiety-like behavior is dependent on the post-ovariectomy time frame in rats. After 12-weeks post ovariectomy rats show high anxiety-like behavior respect to rats at 3-weeks post-ovariectomy in the burying behavior parading. This high anxiety-like behavior is reduced after injection of 1–2 mg/kg diazepam, a typical anxiolytic benzodiazepine drug [23]. Similarly, i.p. injection of 0.5 and 1 mg/kg phytoestrogen genistein (a secondary metabolite obtained from soybeans) significantly reduces anxiety-like behavior in rats at 12-week post-ovariectomy in the light/dark behavioral paradigm through action on the estrogen receptor-β [99, 100]. Additionally, s.c. injection of 0.9 or 0.18 mg/kg genistein exerts similar anxiolytic-like effects in the elevated plus maze than 17β-estradiol in rats subjected to surgical menopausal model. This is consistent with clinical observations that estradiol reduces anxiety symptoms associated with natural and surgical menopause, and additionally supports the potential use of phytoestrogens as an alternative therapy to ameliorate emotional symptoms associated to menopause.

Research in behavioral pharmacology has contributed to the study of pharmacological actions of natural products. In rats at 12-weeks post-ovariectomy, 50 mg/kg by oral rout of the aqueous crude extract of *Montanoa tomentosa*, a Mexican plant traditionally recommended for the treatment of anxiety and other illness of women, reduces anxiety-like behavior in the elevated plus maze [101]. Said actions have been related with pharmacological actions on the $GABA_A$ receptors [102]. Additionally, secondary metabolites from plants, for example, the flavonoids are reported with anxiolytic properties in behavioral models in rats. In this way, 2 and 4 mg/kg, i.p., of the flavonoid chrysin produces anxiolytic-like effects in rats with surgical menopause subjected to the elevated plus maze and the light/dark test [103]; the said effects were produced through action on the $GABA_A$ receptor because the pretreatment with 1 mg/kg picrotoxin, a noncompetitive antagonist of the $GABA_A$ receptor, cancels the anxiolytic-like effect of chrysin.

7. Conclusion

As mentioned before, behavioral pharmacology is an interdisciplinary field. The present chapter tried to reflect briefly the essence of behavioral pharmacology through an anecdotical review of its developments in areas familiar to the authors. All findings mentioned above underline the importance of the research in behavioral pharmacology on the understanding of the neurobiology of different disorders and the mechanism of action of drugs used to treat such disorders, and at the same time, provide a perspective on the current research done in this growing area, which is and will be a cornerstone in the understanding of human behavior and mental health.

Conflict of interest

The authors do not have any conflict of interest.

Author details

Jonathan Cueto-Escobedo[1]*, Fabio García-García[2], Caio Maximino[3] and Juan Francisco Rodríguez-Landa[4]

1 Translational and Clinical Research Department, Institute of Health Sciences, Universidad Veracruzana, Xalapa, México

2 Biomedicine Department, Institute of Health Sciences, Universidad Veracruzana, Xalapa, México

3 Laboratory of Behavioral Neuroscience, Faculty of Psychology, Institute of Health and Biological Studies, Federal University of the South and Southeast of Pará, Marabá, Pará, Brazil

4 Laboratory of Neuropharmacology, Faculty of Biological Pharmaceutical Chemistry, Institute of Neuroethology, Universidad Veracruzana, Xalapa, México

*Address all correspondence to: jcueto@uv.mx

References

[1] Hacker M. History of pharmacology—From antiquity to the twentieth century. In: Pharmacology, Principles and Practice. London: Academic Press; 2009. pp. 1-7

[2] Chast F. A History of Drug Discovery: From First Steps of Chemistry to Achievements in Molecular Pharmacology. London: Academic Press; 2008. pp. 3-62

[3] Stephenson CP, Karanges E, McGregor IS. Trends in the utilization of psychotropic medications in Australia from 2000 to 2011. Australian and New Zealand Journal of Psychiatry. 2013;**47**(1):74-87. DOI: 10.1177/0004867412466595

[4] Sultan RS, Correll CU, Schoenbaum M, King M, Walkup JT, Olfson M. National patterns of commonly prescribed psychotropic medications to young people. Journal of Child and Adolescent Psychopharmacology. 2018;**28**(3):158-165. DOI: 10.1089/cap.2017.0077

[5] Piper BJ, Ogden CL, Simoyan OM, Chung DY, Caggiano JF, Nichols SD, et al. Trends in use of prescription stimulants in the United States and Territories, 2006 to 2016. PLoS One. 2018;**13**(11):e0206100. DOI: 10.1371/journal.pone.0206100

[6] Sluiter MN, de Vries YA, Koning LG, Hak E, Bos JHJ, Schuiling-Veninga CCM, et al. A prescription trend analysis of methylphenidate: Relation to study reports on efficacy. Administration and Policy in Mental Health. 2020;**47**(2):291-299. DOI: 10.1007/s10488-019-00983-6

[7] Wesselhoeft R, Jensen PB, Talati A, Reutfors J, Furu K, Strandberg-Larsen K, et al. Trends in antidepressant use among children and adolescents: A Scandinavian drug utilization study. Acta Psychiatrica Scandinavica. 2020;**141**(1):34-42. DOI: 10.1111/acps.13116

[8] Instituto Nacional de Psiquiatría Ramón de la Fuente Muñiz, Instituto Nacional de Salud Pública, Secretaría de Salud. Encuesta Nacional de Consumo de Drogas, Alcohol y Tabaco 2016-2017: Reporte de Tabaco. México: INPRFM; 2017. Available from: https://encuestas.insp.mx/ena/encodat2017/encodat_tabaco_2016_2017.pdf [Accessed: 26 February 2020]

[9] Bae H, Kerr DCR. Marijuana use trends among college students in states with and without legalization of recreational use: Initial and longer-term changes from 2008 to 2018. Addiction. 2019;**115**:1115-1124. DOI: 10.1111/add.14939

[10] Mihajlov M, Vejmelka L. Internet addiction: A review of the first twenty years. Psychiatria Danubina. 2017;**29**(3):260-272. DOI: 10.24869/psyd.2017.260

[11] Westwater ML, Fletcher PC, Ziauddeen H. Sugar addiction: The state of the science. European Journal of Nutrition. 2016;**55**(Suppl. 2):55-69. DOI: 10.1007/s00394-016-1229-6

[12] Jacques A, Chaaya N, Beecher K, Ali SA, Belmer A, Bartlett S. The impact of sugar consumption on stress driven, emotional and addictive behaviors. Neuroscience and Biobehavioral Reviews. 2019;**103**:178-199. DOI: 10.1016/j.neubiorev.2019.05.021

[13] Branch MN. Behavioral pharmacology. In: Lattal EA, Iversen IH, editors. Experimental Analysis of Behavior. Amsterdam: Elsevier; 1991. pp. 21-70. DOI: 10.1016/j.neubiorev.2019.05.021

[14] Robbins TW, Murphy ER. Behavioural pharmacology: 40+ years of progress, with a focus on glutamate receptors and cognition. Trends in Pharmacological Sciences. 2006;**27**(3):141-148. DOI: 10.1016/j.tips.2006.01.009

[15] Marr MJ. Behavioral pharmacology: Issues of reductionism and causality. In: Barrett JE, Thompson T, Dews P, editors. Advances in Behavioral Pharmacology. Vol. 7. Hillsdale: Lawrence Erlbaum; 1990. pp. 1-12

[16] Branch MN. How research in behavioral pharmacology informs behavioral science. Journal of the Experimental Analysis of Behavior. 2006;**85**(3):407-423. DOI: 10.1901/jeab.2006.130-04

[17] Selye H. A syndrome produced by diverse nocuous agents. Nature. 1936;**138**:132. DOI: 10.1038/138032a0

[18] Pivik RT, Zarcone V, Dement WC, Hollister LE. Delta-9-tetrahydrocannabinol and synhexl: Effects on human sleep patterns. Clinical Pharmacology and Therapeutics. 1972;**13**(3):426-435. DOI: 10.1002/cpt1972133426

[19] Porsolt RD, Le Pichon M, Jalfre M. Depression: A new animal model sensitive to antidepressant treatment. Nature. 1977;**266**(5604):730-732. DOI: 10.1038/266730a0

[20] Pellow S, File SE. Anxiolytic and anxiogenic drug effects on exploratory activity in an elevated plus-maze: A novel test of anxiety in the rat. Pharmacology, Biochemistry, and Behavior. 1986;**24**:525-529. DOI: 10.1016/0091-3057(86)90552-6

[21] Bastuji H, Jouvet M. Successful treatment of idiopathic hypersomnia and narcolepsy with modafinil. Progress in Neuropsychopharmacology and Biological Psychiatry. 1988;**12**(5):695-700. DOI: 10.1016/0278-5846(88)90014-0

[22] Gerrits M, Grootkarijn A, Bekkering BF, Bruinsma M, Den Boer JA, Ter Horst GJ. Cyclic estradiol replacement attenuates stress-induced c-Fos expression in the PVN of ovariectomized rats. Brain Research Bulletin. 2005;**67**(1-2):147-155. DOI: 10.1016/j.brainresbull.2005.06.021

[23] Picazo O, Estrada-Camarena E, Hernández-Aragon A. Influence of the post-ovariectomy time frame on the experimental anxiety and the behavioural actions of some anxiolytic agents. European Journal of Pharmacology. 2006;**530**(1-2):88-94. DOI: 10.1016/j.ejphar.2005.11.024

[24] Kuriyama A, Tabata H. Suvorexant for the treatment of primary insomnia: A systematic review and meta-analysis. Sleep Medicine Reviews. 2017;**35**:1-7. DOI: 10.1016/j.smrv.2016.09.004

[25] Puga-Olguín A, Rodríguez-Landa JF, Rovirosa-Hernández MJ, Germán-Ponciano LJ, Caba M, Meza E, et al. Long-term ovariectomy increases anxiety- and despair-like behaviors associated with lower Fos immunoreactivity in the lateral septal nucleus in rats. Behavioral Brain Research. 2019;**360**:185-195. DOI: 10.1016/j.bbr.2018.12.017

[26] Levitis DA, Lidicker WZ, Freund G. Behavioural biologists don't agree on what constitutes behaviour. Animal Behaviour. 2009;**78**(1):103-110. DOI: 10.1016/j.anbehav.2009.03.018

[27] Bergner RM. What is behavior? And so what? New Ideas in Psychology. 2011;**29**(2):147-155. DOI: 10.1016/j.newideapsych.2010.08.001

[28] Bourin M. Experimental anxiety model for anxiety disorders: Relevance to drug discovery. In: Kim YK, editor. Anxiety Disorders. Advances in

Experimental Medicine and Biology. Singapore: Springer; 2020. pp. 169-184

[29] Planchez B, Surget A, Belzung C. Animal models of major depression: Drawbacks and challenges. Journal of Neural Transmission. 2019;**126**(11):1383-1408. DOI: 10.1016/j.neurol.2015.07.011

[30] Szechtman H, Ahmari SE, Beninger RJ, Eilam D, Harvey BH, Edemann-Callesen H, et al. Obsessive-compulsive disorder: Insights from animal models. Neuroscience and Biobehavioral Reviews. 2017;**76**:254-279. DOI: 10.1016/j.neubiorev.2016.04.019

[31] Gubellini P, Kachidian P. Animal models of Parkinson's disease: An updated overview. Revue Neurologique. 2015;**171**(11):750-761. DOI: 10.1016/j.neurol.2015.07.011

[32] Löscher W. Animal models of seizures and epilepsy: Past, present, and future role for the discovery of antiseizure drugs. Neurochemical Research. 2017;**42**(7):1873-1888. DOI: 10.1007/s11064-017-2222-z

[33] Kuhn BN, Kalivas PW, Bobadilla AC. Understanding addiction using animal models. Frontiers in Behavioral Neuroscience. 2019;**13**:262. DOI: 10.3389/fnbeh.2019.00262

[34] Toth LA, Bhargava P. Animal models of sleep disorders. Comparative Medicine. 2013;**63**(2):91-104

[35] Pearlstein TB. Hormones and depression: What are the facts about premenstrual syndrome, menopause, and hormone replacement therapy? American Journal of Obstetrics and Gynecology. 1995;**173**(2):646-653. DOI: 10.1016/0002-9378(95)90297-x

[36] Maeng LY, Milad MR. Sex differences in anxiety disorders: Interactions between fear, stress, and gonadal hormones. Hormones and Behavior. 2015;**76**:106-117. DOI: 10.1016/j.yhbeh.2015.04.002

[37] Maximino C, Silva RXC, da Silva SNS, Rodrigues LSDS, Barbosa H, de Carvalho TS, et al. Non-mammalian models in behavioral neuroscience: Consequences for biological psychiatry. Frontiers in Behavioral Neuroscience. 2015;**9**:233. DOI: 10.3389/fnbeh.2015.00233

[38] Koebele SV, Bimonte-Nelson HA. Modeling menopause: The utility of rodents in translational behavioral endocrinology research. Maturitas. 2016;**87**:5-17. DOI: 10.1016/j.maturitas.2016.01.015

[39] Atkin T, Comai S, Gobbi G. Drugs for insomnia beyond benzodiazepines: Pharmacology, clinical applications, and discovery. Pharmacological Reviews. 2018;**70**(2):197-245. DOI: 10.1124/pr.117.014381

[40] McEwen BS. Hormones and behavior and the integration of brain-body science. Hormones and Behavior. 2019;**119**:104619. DOI: 10.1016/j.yhbeh.2019.104619

[41] Lamb YN. Pitolisant: A review in narcolepsy with or without cataplexy. CNS Drugs. 2020;**34**:207-218. DOI: 10.1007/s40263-020-00703-x

[42] Willner P. Methods for assessing the validity of animal models of human psychopathology. In: Boulton AA, Baker GB, Martin-Iverson MT, editors. Animal Models in Psychiatry. Clifton: Humana Press; 1991. pp. 1-23

[43] Maximino C, Arndt SS, van der Staay FJ. Animal models. In: Vonk J, Schackelford TK, editors. Encyclopedia of Animal Cognition and Behavior. Basel: Springer Nature Switzerland; 2019. pp. 1-17

[44] Maximino C, van der Staay FJ. Behavioral models in psychopathology:

Epistemic and semantic considerations. Behavioral and Brain Functions. 2019;**15**:1

[45] Belzung C, Lemoine M. Criteria of validity for animal models of psychiatric disorders: Focus on anxiety disorders and depression. Biology of Mood & Anxiety Disorders. 2011;**1**:9

[46] Ferreira GS, Veening-Griffioen D, Boon W, Moors E, Gispen-de Wied C, Schellekens H, et al. A standardized framework to identify optimal animal models for efficacy assessment in drug development. PLoS One. 2019;**14**(6):e0218014. DOI: 10.1371/journal.pone.0218014

[47] Maximino C, De Brito TM, Gouveia A Jr. Construct validity of behavioral models of anxiety: Where experimental psychopathology meets ecology and evolution. Psychology & Neuroscice. 2010;**3**(1):117-123. DOI: 10.3922/j.psns.2010.1.015

[48] Montgomery KC. The relation between fear induced by novel stimulation and exploratory behavior. Journal of Comparative and Physiological Psychology. 1955;**47**: 254-260. DOI: 10.1037/h0043788

[49] Treit D, Menard J, Royan C. Anxiogenic stimuli in the elevated plus-maze. Pharmacology, Biochemistry, and Behavior. 1993;**44**:463-469. DOI: 10.1016/0091-3057(93)90492-c

[50] Bakshi VP, Kalin NH. Animal models and endophenotypes of anxiety and stress disorders. In: Davis KL, Charney D, Coyle JT, Nemeroff C, editors. Neuropsychopharmacology: The Fifth Generation of Progress. New York: American College of Neuropsychopharmacology; 2002. pp. 883-900

[51] Steimer T. Animal models of anxiety disorders in rats and mice: Some conceptual issues. Dialogues in Clinical Neuroscice. 2011;**13**:495-506

[52] Hånell A, Marklund N. Structured evaluation of rodent behavioral tests used in drug discovery research. Frontiers in Behavioral Neuroscience. 2014;**8**:252. DOI: 10.3389/fnbeh.2014.00252

[53] Griebel G, Holmes A. 50 years of hurdles and hope in anxiolytic drug discovery. Nature Reviews. Drug Discovery. 2013;**12**:667-687. DOI: 10.1038/nrd407

[54] Stewart AM, Ullmann JFP, Norton WHJ, Parker MO, Brennan CH, Gerlai R, et al. Molecular psychiatry of zebrafish. Molecular Psychiatry. 2015;**20**:2-17. DOI: 10.1038/mp.2014.128

[55] Fields S, Johnston M. Whither model organism research? Science. 2005;**307**(5717):1885-1886

[56] Black MC. Routes of administration for chemical agents. In: Ostrander GK, editor. The Laboratory Fish. San Diego, CA: Academic Press; 2000. pp. 529-542

[57] De Tolla LJ, Srinivas S, Whitaker BR, Andrews C, Hecker B, Kane AS, et al. Guidelines for the care and use of fish in research. ILAR Journal. 1995;**37**:159-173. DOI: 10.1093/ilar.37.4.159

[58] Zang L, Morikane D, Shimada Y, Tanaka T, Nishimura N. A novel protocol for the oral administration of test chemicals to adult zebrafish. Zebrafish. 2011;**8**:203-210. DOI: 10.1089/zeb.2011.0726

[59] Maximino C, De Brito TM, Dias CAGDM, Gouveia A Jr, Morato S. Scototaxis as anxiety-like behavior in fish. Nature Protocols. 2010;**5**:209-216. DOI: 10.1038/nprot.2009.225

[60] Bencan Z, Sledge D, Levin ED. Buspirone, chlordiazepoxide and diazepam effects in a zebrafish model of

anxiety. Pharmacology, Biochemistry, and Behavior. 2009;**94**:75-80

[61] Maximino C, Benzecry R, Matos KRO, Batista E de JO, Herculano AM, Rosemberg DB, et al. A comparison of the light/dark and novel tank tests in zebrafish. Behaviour. 2012;**149**:1099-1123. DOI: 10.1163/1568539X-00003029

[62] do Nascimento JET, de Morais SM, de Lisboa DS, de Oliveira-Sousa M, Santos SAAR, Magalhães FEA, et al. The orofacial antinociceptive effect of Kaempferol-3-O-rutinoside, isolated from the plant *Ouratea fieldingiana*, on adult zebrafish (*Danio rerio*). Biomedicine & Pharmacotherapy. 2018;**107**:1030-1036. DOI: 10.1016/j.biopha.2018.08.089

[63] dos Santos Sampaio TI, de Melo NC, de Freitas Paiva BT, da Silva Aleluia GA, da Silva Neto FLP, da Silva HR, et al. Leaves of *Spondias mombin* L. a traditional anxiolytic and antidepressant: Pharmacological evaluation on zebrafish (*Danio rerio*). Journal of Ethnopharmacology. 2018;**224**:563-578. DOI: 10.1016/j.jep.2018.05.037

[64] Maximino C, Puty B, Benzecry R, Araújo J, Gomez-Lima M, de Jesus Oliveira Batista E, et al. Role of serotonin in zebrafish (*Danio rerio*) anxiety: Relationship with serotonin levels and effect of buspirone, WAY 100635, SB 224289, fluoxetine and para-chlorophenylalanine (pCPA) in two behavioral models. Neuropharmacology. 2013;**71**:83-97. DOI: 10.1016/j.neuropharm.2013.03.006

[65] Braida D, Donzelli A, Martucci R, Capurro V, Busnelli M, Chini B, et al. Neurohypophysealhormonesmanipulation modulate social and anxiety-related behavior in zebrafish. Psychopharmacology. 2012;**220**:319-330. DOI: 10.1007/s00213-011-2482-2

[66] Choi J-H, Jeong Y-M, Kim S, Lee B, Ariyasiri K, Kim H-T, et al. Targeted knockout of a chemokine-like gene increases anxiety and fear responses. Proceedings of the National Academy of Sciences of the United States of America. 2018;**115**(5):1041-1050. DOI: 10.1073/pnas.1707663115

[67] Amir-Zilberstein L, Blechman J, Sztainberg Y, Norton WHJ, Reuveny A, Borodovsky N, et al. Homeodomain protein Otp and activity-dependent splicing modulate neuronal adaptation to stress. Neuron. 2012;**73**:279-291. DOI: 10.1016/j.neuron.2011.11.019

[68] Mathuru AS, Jesuthasan S. The medial habenula as a regulator of anxiety in adult zebrafish. Frontiers in Neural Circuits. 2013;7:99. DOI: 10.3389/fncir.2013.00099

[69] Kokel D, Peterson RT. Chemobehavioural phenomics and behaviour-based psychiatric drug discovery in the zebrafish. Briefings in Functional Genomics. 2008;7(6):483-490. DOI: 10.1093/bfgp/eln040

[70] Kokel D, Bryan J, Laggner C, White R, Cheung CYJ, Mateus R, et al. Rapid behavior-based identification of neuroactive small molecules in the zebrafish. Natural Chemical Biology. 2010;**6**(3):231-237. DOI: 10.1038/nchembio.307

[71] Bruni G, Rennekamp AJ, Velenich A, McCarroll M, Gendelev L, Fertsch E, et al. Zebrafish behavioral profiling identifies multitarget antipsychotic-like compounds. Natural Chemical Biology. 2016;**12**:559-566. DOI: 10.1038/nchembio.2097

[72] Kozol RA, Abrams AJ, James DM, Buglo E, Yan Q, Dallman JE. Function over form: Modeling groups of inherited neurological conditions in zebrafish. Frontiers in Molecular Neuroscience. 2016;**9**:55. DOI: 10.3389/fnmol.2016.00055

[73] Grone BP, Qu T, Baraban SC. Behavioral comorbidities and drug treatments in a zebrafish scn1lab model of Dravet syndrome. eNeuro. 2017;**4**:ENEURO.0066-17.2017. DOI: 10.1523/ENEURO.0066-17.2017

[74] Sourbron J, Schneider H, Kecskés A, Liu Y, Buening EM, Lagae L, et al. Serotonergic modulation as effective treatment for Dravet syndrome in a zebrafish mutant model. ACS Chemical Neuroscience. 2016;7:588-598. DOI: 10.1021/acschemneuro.5b00342

[75] Sateia MJ, Buysse DJ, Krystal AD, Neubauer DN, Heald JL. Clinical practice guideline for the pharmacologic treatment of chronic insomnia in adults: An American Academy of Sleep Medicine Clinical Practice guideline. Journal of Clinical Sleep Medicine. 2017;**13**(2):307-349. DOI: 10.5664/jcsm.6470

[76] Zammit GK, Weiner J, Damato N, Sillup GP, McMillan CA. Quality of life in people with insomnia. Sleep. 1999;**22**(Suppl. 2):S379-S385

[77] Wickwire EM, Shaya FT, Scharf SM. Health economics of insomnia treatments: The return on investment for a good night's sleep. Sleep Medicine Reviews. 2016;**30**:72-82. DOI: 10.1016/j.smrv.2015.11.004

[78] Ohayon MM. Epidemiology of insomnia: What we know and what we still need to learn. Sleep Medicine Reviews. 2002;**6**:97-111. DOI: 10.1053/smrv.2002.0186

[79] Stahl S. Stahl's Essential Psychopharmacology, Neuroscientific Basis and Practical Applications, Applications. 3rd ed. New York: Cambridge University Press; 2008

[80] Soldatos CR, Dikeos DG, Whitehead A. Tolerance and rebound insomnia with rapidly eliminated hypnotics: A meta-analysis of sleep laboratory studies. International Clinical Psychopharmacology. 1999;**14**(5):287-303

[81] Ashton H. The diagnosis and management of benzodiazepine dependence. Current Opinion in Psychiatry. 2005;**18**(3):249-255. DOI: 10.1097/01.yco.0000165594.60434.84

[82] Everitt H, Baldwin DS, Stuart B, Lipinska G, Mayers A, Malizia AL, et al. Antidepressants for insomnia in adults. Cochrane Database Systemic Reviews. 2018;**5**:CD010753. DOI: 10.1002/14651858.CD010753.pub2

[83] Estivill E, de la Fuente V. Eficacia del ropinirol como tratamiento del insomnio crónico secundario al síndrome de piernas inquietas: datos polisomnográficos. Revista de Neurologia. 1999;**29**:805-807. DOI: 10.33588/rn.2909.99317

[84] Herring WJ, Connor KM, Ivgy-May N, Snyder E, Liu K, Snavely DB, et al. Suvorexant in patients with insomnia: Results from two 3-month randomized controlled clinical trials. Biological Psychiatry. 2016;**79**:136-148. DOI: 10.1016/j.biopsych.2014.10.003

[85] Kuriyama A, Honda M, Hayashino Y. Ramelteon for the treatment of insomnia in adults: A systematic review and meta-analysis. Sleep Medicine. 2014;**15**:385-392. DOI: 10.1016/j.sleep.2013.11.788

[86] Sys J, Van Cleynenbreugel S, Deschodt M, Van der Linden L, Tournoy J. Efficacy and safety of non-benzodiazepine and non-Z-drug hypnotic medication for insomnia in older people: A systematic literature review. European Journal of Clinical Pharmacology. 2020;**76**:363-381. DOI: 10.1007/s00228-019-02812-z

[87] De la Herrán-Arita AK, García-García F. Current and emerging options

for the drug treatment of narcolepsy. Drugs. 2013;**73**(16):1771-1781. DOI: 10.1007/s40265-013-0127-y

[88] Leu-Semenescu S, Nittur N, Golmard JL, Arnulf I. Effects of Pitolisant, a histamine H3 inverse agonist, in drug-resistant idiopathic and symptomatic hypersomnia: A chart review. Sleep Medicine. 2014;**15**(6):681-687. DOI: 10.1016/j.sleep.2014.01.021

[89] Lin JS, Dauvilliers Y, Arnulf I, Bastuji H, Anaclet C, Parmentier R, et al. An inverse agonist of the histamine H(3) receptor improves wakefulness in narcolepsy: Studies in orexin$^{-/-}$ mice and patients. Neurobiology of Disease. 2008;**30**(1):74-83. DOI: 10.1016/j.nbd.2007.12.003

[90] Ashworth S, Berges A, Rabiner EA, Wilson AA, Comley RA, Lay RYK, et al. Unexpectedly high affinity of a novel histamine H(3) receptor antagonist, GSK239512, in vivo in human brain, determined using PET. British Journal of Pharmacology. 2014;**171**(5):1241-1249. DOI: 10.1111/bph.12505

[91] Passani MB, Lin JS, Hancock A, Crochet S, Blandina P. The histamine H3 receptor as a novel therapeutic target for cognitive and sleep disorders. Trends in Pharmacological Sciences. 2004;**25**(12):618-625. DOI: 10.1016/j.tips.2004.10.003

[92] Martínez-Mota L. Sexual hormones and mental health. Salud Mental. 2020;**43**(1):1-2. DOI: 10.17711/SM.0185-3325.2020.001

[93] Paoletti AM, Floris S, Mannias M, Orru M, Crippa D, Orlandi R, et al. Evidence that cyproterone acetate improves psychological symptoms and enhances the activity of the dopaminergic system in postmenopause. The Journal of Clinical Endocrinology and Metabolism. 2001;**86**(2):608-612. DOI: 10.1210/jcem.86.2.7179

[94] Taylor M. Psychological consequences of surgical menopause. Journal of Reproductive Medicine. 2001;**46**(Suppl. 3):317-324

[95] Muttukrishna S, Sharma S, Barlow DH, Ledger W, Groome N, Sathanandan M. Serum inhibins, estradiol, progesterone and FSH in surgical menopause: A demonstration of ovarian pituitary feedback loop in women. Human Reproduction. 2002;**17**(10):2535-2539. DOI: 10.1093/humrep/17.10.2535

[96] Kalu DN. The ovariectomized rat model of postmenopausal bone loss. Bone and Mineral. 1991;**15**(3):175-191. DOI: 10.1016/0169-6009(91)90124-I

[97] Bossé R, Di Paolo T. The modulation of brain dopamine and $GABA_A$ receptors by estradiol: A clue for CNS changes occurring at menopause. Cellular and Molecular Neurobiology. 1996;**16**(2):199-212. DOI: 10.1007/bf02088176

[98] Rodríguez-Landa JF, Cueto-Escobedo J. Introductory chapter: A multidisciplinary look at menopause. In: Rodríguez-Landa JF, Cueto-Escobedo J, editors. A Multidisciplinary Look at Menopause. Rijeka: Intech; 2017. pp. 1-5. DOI: 10.5772/intechopen.70114

[99] Rodríguez-Landa JF, Hernández-Figueroa JD, Hernández-Calderón BC, Saavedra M. Anxiolytic-like effect of phytoestrogen genistein in rats with long-term absence of ovarian hormones in the black and white model. Progress in Neuropsychopharmacology and Biological Psychiatry. 2009;**33**(2):367-372. DOI: 10.1016/j.pnpbp.2008.12.024

[100] Rodríguez-Landa JF, Hernández-López F, Saavedra M. Involvement of estrogen receptors in the anxiolytic-like effect of phytoestrogen genistein in rats with 12-weeks postovariectomy. Pharmacology and

Pharmacy. 2012;**3**(4):439-446. DOI: 10.4236/pp.2012.3405

[101] Rodríguez-Landa JF, Rodríguez-Santiago MG, Rovirosa-Hernández MJ, García-Orduña F, Carro-Juárez M. Aqueous crude extract of *Montanoa tomentosa* exerts anxiolytic-like effects in female rats with long-term absence of ovarian hormones. Journal of Chemical, Biological and Physical Sciences. 2014;**4**(5):37-46. DOI: 10.1177/2515690X18762953

[102] Estrada-Camarena E, Sollozo-Dupont I, Islas-Preciado D, González-Trujano ME, Carro-Juárez M, López-Rubalcava C. Anxiolytic- and anxiogenic-like effects of *Montanoa tomentosa* (Asteraceae): Dependence on the endocrine condition. Journal of Ethnopharmacology. 2019;**241**:112006. DOI: 10.1016/j.jep.2019.112006

[103] Rodríguez-Landa JF, Hernández-López F, Cueto-Escobedo J, Herrera-Huerta EV, Rivadeneyra-Domínguez E, Bernal-Morales B, et al. Chrysin (5,7-dihydroxyflavone) exerts anxiolytic-like effects through $GABA_A$ receptors in a surgical menopause model in rats. Biomedicine & Pharmacotherapy. 2019;**109**:2387-2395. DOI: 10.1016/j.biopha.2018.11.111

Chapter 3

Berry Supplementation and Their Beneficial Effects on Some Central Nervous System Disorders

Fernández-Demeneghi Rafael, Vargas-Moreno Isidro, Acosta-Mesa Héctor-Gabriel, Puga-Olguín Abraham, Campos-Uscanga Yolanda, Romo-González Tania, Guzmán-Gerónimo Rosa-Isela, Patraca-Camacho Lorena and Herrera-Meza Socorro

Abstract

This chapter is based in the compilation and analysis of different in vitro, preclinical, and clinical studies, which explored the potential beneficial bioactivity of supplementation with berries on some alterations in the central nervous system (CNS). The last section of the chapter describes the possible mechanisms of action of polyphenols, anthocyanins, and other compounds present in berries as well as their relationship with anxiety, depression, and Alzheimer's (AD) and Parkinson's diseases (PD) and their implication in the prevention of cognitive decline and senescence motor functions. Electronic databases as Springer, PubMed, Scopus, and Elsevier were used. Papers were selected by topic specially those related with berries, year of publication, and authors. The present chapter evidenced the potential health effect as neuroprotector of different berries and their bioactive compounds mainly flavonoids, polyphenols, and anthocyanins, on diseases such as anxiety, depression, and Alzheimer's and Parkinson's diseases. In conclusion, for human nutrition berry fruit supplementation might be an excellent source of antioxidant and alternative for prevention and reduction of symptoms in diseases such as anxiety, depression, Alzheimer's, and Parkinson's.

Keywords: berry, anthocyanins, polyphenols, neuroprotection, prevention

1. Introduction

Berries with a high antioxidant activity have drawn the attention of scientists due to their potential antioxidant, anticancer, anti-inflammatory, and neuroprotective-related effects, identified in in vivo studies [1]. It is well established that many species of berries, for example, strawberries (*Fragaria ananassa*), blueberries (*Vaccinium corymbosum*), raspberries (*Rubus idaeus*), and blackberries (*Rubus fruticosus*), are rich in bioactive compounds such as flavonoids, polyphenols, and anthocyanins. These compounds could be a supplementation alternative because

IntechOpen

they are able to cross the blood-brain barrier and accumulate in various structures [2, 3] related to learning, memory, cognition process, and modification of behavior. In addition, their anti-neurodegenerative properties have been observed in diseases such as anxiety associated with stressful events [4] and reduction of depression, AD, and PD symptoms. Additionally, an association has been observed between the consumption of berries and increase in dendritic spine density in some brain structures and hippocampal neurogenesis [5]. In this way, the berry consumption and their bioactive compounds (i.e., polyphenols and anthocyanins) might be an excellent alternative for human nutrition when consumed fresh. They can be consumed as yogurt, juice, jam, or like dietary supplements that can be used as functional and nutraceutical foods.

Food is considered as a functional food if, in addition to its basic nutritional, it generates a beneficial effect in the physiological processes in the organism [6]. In the same way, a nutraceutical is a food or part of a food that produces health benefits besides its nutritional content [7, 8]. In the present chapter, we discuss the potential beneficial effects of berries and their derivatives on some central nervous system diseases.

2. Berries

Enhanced consumption of fruits and vegetables is highly recommended in dietary guidelines. Specially, the consumption of berries is recommended due to their antioxidant properties [1]. Berries, in botanical terms, are defined as fleshy fruits that emerge from the plant ovary that encloses the seeds; due to this, berries include grapes, blueberries, black currants, and coffee beans [9].

In this chapter we will focus on strawberries, blueberries, raspberries, chokeberries, black currants, and blackberries, among other endemic fruits. We selected these fruits because, in addition to being rich in polyphenols and anthocyanins, they are the most consumed in human diet; therefore, more studies related to their supplementation and chemical composition have been published.

Berries (i.e., blackberry, black raspberry, blueberry, cranberry, red raspberry, and strawberry) are popularly consumed either fresh, frozen, or processed as yogurts, beverages, jam and jellies, as well as dried or canned. Furthermore, berry extracts have been used as a functional food or dietary supplement [1].

Berries (blueberry, strawberry, blackberry, and Brazilian berries {*Eugenia uniflora L.*}) are considered an important group within functional foods, since multiple investigations have shown that their consumption produces beneficial health effects ranging from the mitigation of adverse physiological processes related to cardiovascular diseases and metabolic disorders to the amelioration of cognitive brain functions [10]. This highlights their ability to modulate neuroinflammation [11], glucoregulation [12], brain vascular function [13], and hippocampal neurogenesis [5]. These effects have been linked to their chemical compounds, specifically, to the presence of phenolic compounds in these fruits [14]. **Table 1** shows specifically most consumed berries, their effect produced, and metabolite involved.

Even though the composition and the content of these compounds are dependent on the plant species, production status, agricultural processing, and storage, berries are an excellent source of polyphenols, flavonoids, and anthocyanins [20, 21], which have been related to their potential beneficial effects on health.

Berry	Effect	Metabolite involved	Ref
Blueberry *(Vaccinium Virgatum A.)*	Antioxidant	Anthocyanins (1202 mg)	[9]
Strawberry *(Fragaria ananassa Duch.)*	Antioxidant	Polyphenols (13550 mg)	[9]
Blackberry *(Rubus sp.)*	Antioxidant	Anthocyanins (870 mg)	[9]
Blueberry *(*NS)*	Modulate neuroinflammation	Flavonoids: various concentrations of blueberry (50-500 μg)	[10]
Blueberry Highbush *(Vaccinium corymbosum)*	Glucoregulation	Anthocyanins-flavonols (220 mg)	[11]
Blueberry *(Vaccinium corybosum)*	Synaptic plasticity	Anthocyanins (10.2 mg)/ Total phenolics (33 mg)	[12]
Blueberry *(*NS)*	Hippocampal neurogenesis	Blueberry extract diet (20 g) (*NS anthocyanins or polyphenols)	[5]
Rasperry *(Rubus idaeus)*	Anti-cancer	Anthocyanins (314 mg)	[14]
Strawberry Beverage *(*NS)*	Anti-inflamatory/ hypoglycemic	Total phenols (94.7 mg)/ Anthocyanins (39 mg)	[15]
Grape (**NS*)	Genoprotective	Anthocyanins (1576.5 mg)/ Total phenolics (2750.4 mg)	[16]
Blueberry Highbush *(Vaccinium corymbosum)*	Neuroprotection/ Proneurogenesis	Anthocyanins (4968·3 ng)	[17]
Cranberry *(Vaccinium oxycoccus)*	Vascular	Polyphenols (835 mg)/ Anthocyanins (94 mg)	[18]
Rabbiteye Blueberry *(Vacciniumn ashei)*	Motor and cognitive function Anxiolytic Genoprotective	Anthocyanins (2.6-3.2 mg)	[19]

NS: not specified; Ref: reference

Table 1.
Berries: effects and metabolites involved.

3. Active metabolites from berries with pharmacological activity

Berries are rich in phytochemicals such as minerals, vitamins, fatty acids, and dietary fibers and specifically contain provitamin A, minerals, vitamin C, and B complex vitamins. Additionally, fruits contain soluble solids, fructose, and chemopreventive agents as A, C, and E vitamins, folic acid, calcium, and selenium. Carotene and lutein are present in berries as well as phytosterols such as sitosterol and stigmasterol and also contain triterpene esters, and there is an excellent source of phenolic molecules such as flavonols, flavanols, proanthocyanidins, ellagitannins, phenolic acids, and anthocyanins specially cyanidin-3-glucoside, gallic acid, pelargonidin, delphinidin, peonidin, and malvidin, among others [22].

The metabolism, bioavailability, and biological effects attributed to berries depend specifically on the type of chemical structure contained in its phenolic compounds that individually or synergistically exert protection against several health disorders [23]. **Table 2** shows the main phytochemical compounds present in berries and their representative chemical structures.

Berry	TP mg/100 g	TA mg/100 g	Characteristic structure	Ref
Blueberry (FW)	711.3 ±	360 ± 0.76	Gallic acid 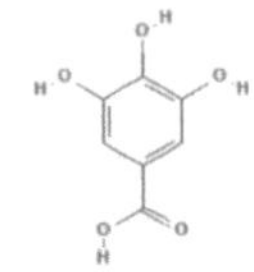	[22]
Blackberry (FW)	2611	104	Gallic acid 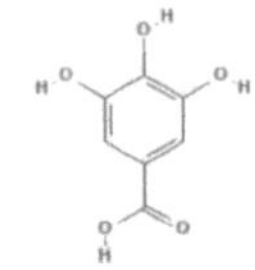	[23]
Cranberry (DW)	59	117	Cyanidin 3-glucoside 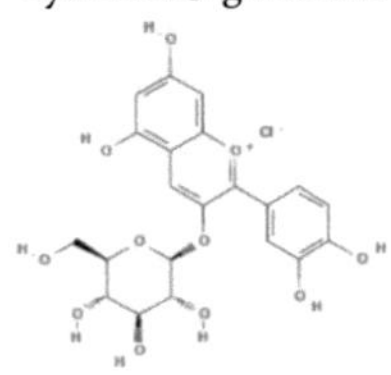	[24]
Raspberry Black Red (FW)	267 234.25	197.2 ± 3.5 68.17 ± 3.02	Cyanidin 3-glucoside 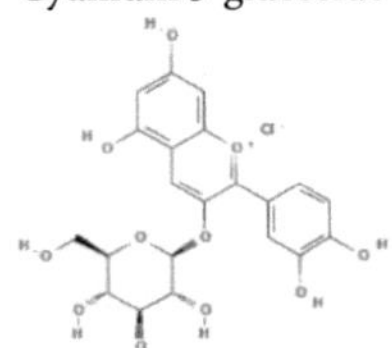	[25]
Blackcurrant (DW)	2382.4 ± 60.8	403.3 ± 11	Cyanidin 3-rutinoside 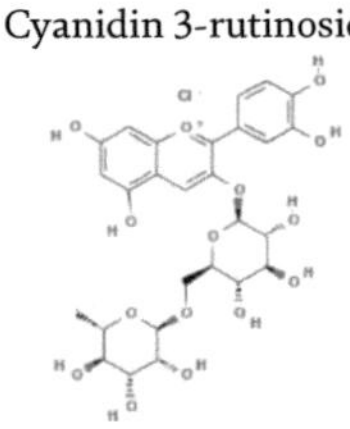	[26]

Chemical structure was determined according to berry bioactive compound. TP: total polyphenols; TF: total flavonoids; TA: total anthocyanins; FW: fresh weight; DW: dry weight.

Table 2.
Total polyphenols, anthocyanins and characteristic structure content of berries.

3.1 Polyphenols

Polyphenols or phenolic compounds are phytochemicals that result from the secondary metabolism of plants coming from the metabolic pathway of shikimic acid and acetate-malonate. They are composed of various chemical structures characterized by an aromatic nucleus of benzene substituted by a hydroxyl group called phenol [21]. Differences between subclasses are given by the number of phenolic rings and the elements attached to them, thus creating several families of compounds, such as flavonoids, anthocyanins, flavones, tannins, and coumarins, among others [21, 27–29].

Polyphenols are present in fruits, vegetables, leaves, nuts, seeds, flowers, and barks [30] and act as inhibitors or activators for a wide variety of mammalian enzyme systems and as metal chelators and oxygen free radical scavengers [31, 32]. Moreover, it has been reported that some flavonoids rise ion chlorine flow at the $GABA_A$ receptor in male rats [33, 34]. They can act as positive or negative modulators by direct actions on the effect of GABA [35, 36]. Considerable scientific evidence has shown that flavonoids are able to cross into the brain and influence brain function [37, 38]. They have a variety of effects like relief of anxiety, antidepressant actions, and neuroprotective [29] and sedative actions [39].

The ability of polyphenols to modulate the activity of different enzymes and consequently interfere in signaling mechanisms and different cellular processes may be due, in part, to the physicochemical characteristics of these compounds, which allow them to participate in different oxide-reduction cellular metabolic reactions [40].

A diet rich in polyphenols has been shown to augment health [41]. It is best known for its biological effects in humans as anti-inflammatory [42] and anticarcinogenic [43]; in vitro as antiviral [44]; and in animals as gastroprotector [45] and antibacterial [46]; among others. More than 8000 phenolic compounds are known in nature [47], which according to their chemical composition are divided into 2 groups: phenolic acids (benzoic and cinnamic) and flavonoids (flavonoids, anthocyanins, and tannins) [48]. For the purposes of this chapter, we will focus on describing flavonoids in a general sense and anthocyanins in a particular manner.

3.2 Flavonoids

Their name derives from the Latin *flavus*, which means "yellow," and constitutes the most abundant subclass of polyphenols within the vegetable kingdom [49]. They are low molecular weight compounds sharing a common diphenylpyrane skeleton (C6-C3-C6′), composed by two phenyl rings (A and B) bound through a heterocyclic pyran C ring. All flavonoids are hydroxylated structures in their aromatic rings and are therefore polyphenolic structures [41].

The main subgroups of flavonoid include flavonols, flavones, flavanones (dihydroflavones), isoflavones, and anthocyanins [50]. The flavonoid quercetin (4 mg/day) produces antineoplastic effects [51] and cholesterol-lowering effects in Japanese women aged 29–79 years old (9.3 ± 7.4 mg/day) [52], and at preclinical research in rats, quercetin (25 and 50 mg/kg) produces antithrombotic effects [53], while a hepatic regenerative effect was detected with supplementations of silymarin (100 mg/kg/day) [54].

Among the most reported effects of flavonoids on the central nervous system are their participation in learning and memory mechanisms in Sprague Dawley rats supplemented with nobiletin (725 mg; extracted from *Citrus depressa* peels) [55]; in vitro aid in the treatment of AD by inhibiting the formation of plaques related to memory loss (myricetin, 1 mM) [56] and their neuroprotective role in PD (quercetin, 0.1 μM, or sesamin, 1 pM) [57]; and in male Swiss mice, antidepressant effect supplemented with *Schinus molle* L. (0.3–3 mg/kg) [58] and anxiolytic activities in Wistar rats (1 mg/kg of chrysin i.p.) and zebra fish (1 98 μL/0.1 g b.w.) [59].

3.3 Anthocyanins

Anthocyanins are an important group of water-soluble flavonoid compounds responsible for the red, purple, and blue colors in flowers, fruits, and other parts of plants that are not toxic for human consumption [48]. Their name derives from the Greek *αυθός* (*anthos*) meaning "flower" and *κυανός* (*kyáneos*) meaning "blue" [60].

They are polyhydroxy- or polymethoxy-glycosides derived from the basic structure, 2-phenyl benzopyryllium [61]. They consist of structures known as anthocyanidins or aglycones, which consist of an aromatic ring attached to a heterocyclic ring containing oxygen which, in turn, is linked to a third aromatic ring. When anthocyanidins are found in glucosylated form, they are then known as anthocyanins and are mainly accompanied by glucose, rhamnose, galactose, arabinose, xylose, and other disaccharides and trisaccharides [62]. These carbohydrates are always bound to anthocyanidin position 3, and glucose is often found additionally in position 5 and, less commonly, in positions 7, 3′, and 4′ [63].

Anthocyanins are less water-soluble than when they are found in glucosinolates and rarely exist in free form in food. Today, about 19 natural anthocyanidins are known, although the most commonly found in foods are six: pelargonidin, delphinidin, cyanidin, petunidin, peonidin, and malvidin [64], names derived from the plant source from which they were first isolated. In the same sense, a measure of the antioxidant capacity of anthocyanin pigments revealed that cyanidin-3-glucoside and delphinidin-3-glucoside have the highest antioxidant activity [65] and have been identified in fruits coming from the berry family [66], specifically in blackberries [67, 68].

It is important to mention that anthocyanins resist passage through the digestive tract of mammals and are absorbed in the stomach and in the middle portion of the small intestine, reaching the bloodstream almost intact [69]; they reach organs such as the liver, eyes, and brain, thus accumulating in them [14, 70].

4. Biological effects

The biological functions of anthocyanins can be classified into two types: those related to their antioxidant capacity and those involved in the modulation of cell signaling pathways [71]. In general, they are attributed with effects such as the prevention and/or reduction of atherosclerosis [72]; reduction in the incidence of cardiovascular disease [73]; anticancer [74] and anti-inflammatory activity [75]; hypoglycemic effects [76]; and augmented visual acuity [77] and cognition [78].

Specifically, anthocyanins cross the blood-brain barrier and accumulate in brain regions related to learning and memory, such as the hippocampus and cerebral cortex, modifying behavior [2]. It has been observed in in vitro studies that consumption of these compounds inhibits the enzyme monoamine oxidase (MAO), in which increased activity is related to AD and other neurological disorders [79]. In addition, they display antioxidant capabilities, such as decreasing free radicals and stress signals controlling calcium homeostasis in the brain [80, 81], as well as the presence of hydrogen peroxide (H_2O_2) and radicals peroxide (ROO) and superoxide (O2) [82, 83]. They also exert protective effects against oxidative stress in cellular models of PD [84] and promote optimal neurotransmission, primarily in advanced age [21].

It has also been observed that anthocyanins ameliorate anti-ocular-inflammatory in male Lewis rats supplemented with crude aronia extract (*Aronia melanocarpa*) in doses of 100 mg/kg, an effect similar to that found in ophthalmic prednisolone in a dose of 10 mg; this effect is evidenced by the direct blockage of the expression of the iNOS and COX-2 enzymes leading to suppression of NO, PGE2, and TNF-α production [85]. Another study in female Wistar rats ovariectomized and supplemented with anthocyanin (200 mg/kg, 7 days of treatment) showed an augment in learning and memory in rats with estrogen deficiency caused by ovariectomy, showing lower errors and latency times in shuttle box test [86].

5. Berries and bioactive compounds on brain diseases

The recent increase in life expectancy worldwide has augmented the incidence of age-related diseases, particularly neurodegenerative diseases and psychiatric disorders.

Below, we will describe the effects of berry consumption and the relationship between diseases such as anxiety, depression, Alzheimer's and Pasrkinson's diseases, as well as human cognition, because those are the most common mental illness and neurodegenerative diseases [5].

In addition, you will find in **Table 3** the most recent research carried out related with supplementation in humans and in animal models and, additionally, study design and summarized findings.

5.1 Anxiety

Anxiety is a common and chronic psychiatric disorder that is a source of suffering and impairment [96]. In 2017, the World Health Organization reported that more than 260 million people suffer from an anxiety disorder [97]. Its pharmacological treatment is based on the use of benzodiazepine drugs, as well as some antidepressants with anxiolytic activity [98]. Unfortunately, these drugs are accompanied by severe side effects such as sedation, pharmacological tolerance, and drug dependence [99, 100]; in this sense, some patients complement their therapies with natural compounds coming from plants.

The study of the potential effect of berries on anxiety, due to their high content of polyphenols and anthocyanins associated with anxiolytic activity at the preclinical level, has attracted important interest [101, 102]. It has been observed that these compounds, present in blueberries, have shown anxiolytic effects in animal models and their possible mechanisms of action are related to the antioxidant properties of anthocyanins [103] which inhibit the enzyme monoamine oxidases (MAOs), decreasing its activity and providing neuroprotection [77, 104].

Supplementation with blueberries in mice for 30 days has shown to increase the time spent in the open arms (anxiolytic effect) in the elevated plus maze test (EPM); in addition, it is shown to reduce oxidative damage to neural DNA, and this antioxidant neural protection has been proposed as a mechanism for the anxiolytic property of berries [19].

One of the most studied berries for anxiety at the preclinical level is the black chokeberry (*Aronia melanocarpa)* belonging to the Rosacea family [105], for example, in male Wistar rats, the acute administration of the juice at doses of 5 and 10 ml/kg exerts dose-dependent anxiolytic activity in the social interaction test in a manner comparable to diazepam [102]. While, subchronic administration of *Aronia melanocarpa* fruit juice (10 ml/kg, orally) in male Wistar rats induces a time-dependent anxiolytic effect [106]. Furthermore, the month-long unlimited consumption of black chokeberry juice (>20 ml/kg b.w daily) exerts reduction of anxiety-like behavior associated with MAO-A/MAO-B inhibitions [104], which is probably due to the high antioxidant activity that black chokeberry has shown to have [107].

On the other hand, this berry fruit has been evaluated in different concentrations and behavioral tests such as the EPM and the social interaction test [102]. Likewise, a methanolic extract of blackberry (*Rubus fruticosus*) was used and reported an anxiolytic effect (100, 200, and 300 mg/kg, orally) in the hole-board test in a dose-dependent response [108]; also, the effect of *Rubus brasiliensis* fruits in Wistar rats has been studied, reporting an anxiolytic effect in EPM, in a dose of 2.5 mg/kg administered per gavage [109]. In turn, an anxiety-related effect has been reported in treated male Swiss mice through supplemented water (2.6–3.2 mg/kg) per day of anthocyanins present in blueberry (*Vaccinium ashei*) [19].

Our working group [4] recently reported the anxiolytic effect from blackberry juice (doses intermediate: 5.83 mg/kg anthocyanins, 27.10 mg/kg polyphenols) on EPM in male Wistar rats, and the design was accompanied by the forced swim test (6 min). A decrease in the anxiety index was observed, without alterations in locomotor activity. This was similar to the group administered with the anxiolytic drug diazepam. Results revealed a better response to behavioral stress in the rats treated with blackberry juice, reinforcing the effects previously reported in EPM (**Table 3**).

The anxiolytic effect of some flavonoids and anthocyanins has been identified by affinity to $GABA_A$ receptors [89, 110]. However, its antioxidant capacity is still

Topic	Author/ location	Study design	Intervention	Summarized findings
Anxiety	Fernández-Demeneghi *et al.*, 2019 [4]/ Mexico	n=45, 21 days treatment, Wistar male rats (200- 250 g)	Five groups were used: Veh (control group administered with 8.7 ml/kg), BL (low dose group of blackberry juice, 2.6 mg/kg of anthocyanins, 14.57 mg/ kg of polyphenols) BM (medium dose group of blackberry juice, 5.83 mg/ kg anthocyanins, 27.10 mg/kg polyphenols) BH (high-dose blackberry juice group 10.57 mg/kg anthocyanins, 38.4 mg/kg polyphenols) DZP (diazepam group administered 2 mg/kg).	The intermediate dose of blackberry juice (5.83 mg/kg of anthocyanins, 27.10 mg / kg of polyphenols) had an anxiolytic effect similar to DZP, improving coping strategies at the behavioral level. These results were supplemented by the forced swim test, where medium and high doses improved the response to acute stress.
Depression	Chang *et al.*, 2016 [85]/ USA-UK	n=82643 women. Prospectively, the study examined the associations between the estimated usual intake of flavonoids in the diet and the risk of depression. Semiquantitative food frequency questionnaire was applied (FFQ).	Two samples were used: Nurses' Health Study (NHSI) (from 1976 nurses aged 30-55) and NHSII (from 1989 nurses aged 25-42).	Higher flavonoid intakes may be associated with lower depression risk, particularly among older women.
	Khalid *et al.*, 2017 [86]/United Kingdom	n=21 university students (18-21 years)/ The Positive and Negative Affect Schedule-NOW (PANAS-NOW) was used to assess current mood.	Two groups were used: The flavonoid-rich wild blueberry (WBB), which administered 253 mg of anthocyanins, a combination of 30 g of lyophilized WBB, 30 ml of Rocks Orange Squash and 220 ml of water), placebo (4 mg of WBB, 30 ml of Rocks Orange Squash and 220 ml of water were combined).	In both studies, an increase in positive affection was observed after 2 hours of consumption of the WBB drink. Flavonoid supplementation can play a key role in promoting positive mood and are a possible way to prevent dysphoria and depression.
		n=50 children (7-10)/child version of the Positive and Negative Affect Scale (PANAS-C).	Two groups were used: The flavonoid-rich wild blueberry (WBB) 253 mg anthocyanins, combination of 30 g lyophilized WBB, 30 ml Rocks Orange Squash and 170 ml water); placebo (4 mg WBB, 30 ml Rocks Orange Squash and 170 ml water were combined).	
	Nabavi *et al.*, 2018 [87]/Iran	n=40, 7 days treatment, balb/c strain mice (5 weeks old, 20-25 g).	Four groups were used: control (healthy group), BCCAO (group with bilateral occlusion of the common carotid artery) 10 mg/kg (group with lesion + 10 mg/kg of aqueous extract of red berries of *H. Androsaemum* (WE) 30 mg/kg (group with lesion + 30 mg/kg of WE).	The protective effects of WE in post-stroke depression in a mouse model were demonstrated *in vivo*, both groups administered with WE reduced immobility time in forced swim and tail suspension tests. These findings are correlated with the antioxidant capacity of its bioactive constituents.
	Di Lorenzo *et al*, 2019 [88]/Italy	n=50, 7 days treatment i.p., balb/c strain mice (2 weeks old, 20-25 g).	Five groups were used: 1) control: healthy group, 2) BCCAO (group with stroke common carotid artery bilateral occlusion), 3) 25 mg/kg (lesion + 25 mg/kg Maqui berry extract (MBE)), 4) 50 mg/kg (lesion + 50 mg/kg MBE), 5) 100 mg/kg (lesion + 100 mg/kg MBE).	The results showed that the antidepressant-like activity provided by the extract, which was found to restore normal mouse behavior in both despair swimming and tail suspension tests, could be linked to its antioxidant activity, leading to the conclusion that maqui berries might be useful for supporting pharmacological therapy of Post-stroke depression by modulating oxidative stress.

Topic	Author/ location	Study design	Intervention	Summarized findings
Alzheimer's disease	Gutierres *et al.*, 2014 [89]/Brazil	Male Wistar rats (3-months-1-year-old, 350-400g), 7 days of treatment with 200 mg/kg anthocyanin (ANT) the rats were injected with intracerebroventricular streptozotocin (3 mg/kg) (STZ), and four days later the behavior parameters were performed.	Four different groups: control (CTRL), anthocyanin (ANT), streptozotocin (STZ) and streptozotocin + anthocyanin (STZ + ANT).	A memory deficit was found in the STZ group, but ANT treatment showed that it prevents this impairment of memory. This work demonstrated that anthocyanin is able to regulate ion pump activity and cholinergic neurotransmission, as well as being able to enhance memory and act as an anxiolytic compound in animals with sporadic dementia of Alzheimer's type.
	McNamara *et al*, 2018 [90]/USA	n=76, 24 weeks treatment, study conducted in men and women aged 62-80 with cognitive impairment. They used the Dysexecutive Questionnaire.	Four groups were used: FO (fish oil + placebo powder), BB (blueberry [*Vaccinium sp*] powder + placebo oil), FO+BB (fish oil + cranberry powder), PL (oil + placebo powder). Fish oil (400 mg EPA (1.6 g) and 200 mg DHA (0.8 g)) and cranberry powder (phenolic concentration (20.4±0.31), anthocyanins (14.5±0.04)).	It was demonstrated that supplementation with FO and BB showed a reduction of self-reported inefficiencies in daily operation, by the BB group showed less interference in memory.
Parkinson's Disease	Fan *et al.*, 2018 [91]/ New Zealand	n= 11 male patients with Parkinson's disease and older than 40 years old. 2 sessions where samples of plasma and cerebrospinal fluid (CSF) were taken (in both sessions a 12-hour low anthocyanin diet was requested before taking the samples).	Study of pre and post treatment samples, where patients were supplemented with 300 mg blackcurrant capsules (35% anthocyanins, Super Currantex® 20) twice daily for four weeks.	The neuropeptide cyclic glycine protein (cGP), a natural BCA nutrient, was shown to be effectively absorbed in the brain after supplementation. The increase of cyclic glycine proline (cGP) in plasma and cephalorachidian fluid in Parkison patients is mainly due to central uptake of the neuropeptide in plasma. Thus, the role of insulin-like growth factor 1 (IGF-1) improves in patients with Parkinson's disease.
	Qian *et al.*, 2019 [92]/ China	n=45, 3 weeks treatment, 6-week old male C57BL/6 mice (18-22 g). This study was designed to investigate the effects of the ANC rich blueberry extracts (BBE) on behavior and oxidative stress in the mouse model of PD induced by 1- methyl-4-phenyl-1,2,3,6- tetrahydropyridine (MPTP).	Five groups were used: 1) control (received i.p. saline), 2) MPTP (received i.p. MPTP 30 mg/kg for 5 days and saline, 3)BBE 50 mg/kg (received i.p. MPTP 30 mg/kg for 5 days and 50 mg/kg blueberry extract (BBE), 4) BBE 100 mg/kg (received i.p. MPTP 30 mg/kg for 5 days and 100 mg/kg of BBE) and 5) i.p MPTP and fed daily with levodopa and benserazide (10 mg/kg/day).	BBE improved motor function in MPTP- induced Parkinson's mice through a possible mechanism of their antioxidant capacity to eliminate free radicals and reduce oxidative damage to neurons.

Topic	Author/ location	Study design	Intervention	Summarized findings
Other effects	Devore *et al.*, 2012 [93]/USA	n=16,010 women, aged ≥70; follow-up assessments were conducted twice, at two-year intervals.	Follow-up questionnaire on eating habits (2-year period) and assessment of congenital impairment. Six cognitive tests were administered: Telephone Interview of Cognitive Status, a telephone adaptation of the Mini-Mental State Examination; East Boston Memory Test – immediate and delayed recalls; category fluency; delayed recall of the Telephone Interview of Cognitive Status 10- word list; and backwards digit span.	Increased consumption of berries and anthocyanidins, as well as total flavonoids, was shown to be associated with slower progression of cognitive impairment in older women.
	Watson *et al.*, 2015 [94]/New Zealand	n=36 healthy, young participants (18-35 years). The battery used was formed: digit vigilance, stroop, rapid visual information processing (RVIP) and logical reasoning.	Three intervention drinks were used: 1. control (containing 0 mg polyphenols), 2. Blackadder (7.78 mg/kg anthocyanins from an extract of Ribes nigrum). 3. DelCyan (trademark) (8.05 mg/kg anthocyanins from a blackcurrant extract).	It was demonstrated that the consumption of drinks supplemented with blackcurrants produce a cognitive benefit in healthy young people, evidenced by greater accuracy in the RIVP test; likewise, Blackadder improved reaction times in the task of monitoring digits. Clinically significant inhibition of monoamine oxidase-B and monoamine oxidase-A was identified using a commonly consumed fruit.
	Whyte & Williams (2015) [95]/United Kingdom	n=16 children (8-10 years), 7 days of treatment. Two hours after consumption, the children completed a battery of five cognitive tests comprising the Go-NoGo, Stroop, Rey's Auditory Verbal Learning Task, Object Location Task, and a Visual N-back.	Two intervention drinks were used: 1. blueberry (prepared by mixing 200 g of Star variety blueberries with 100 ml, which contained 143 mg of anthocyanins). Control (combined with blueberry drink for sugars and vitamin C by adding 0.02 g of vitamin C powder, 8.22 g of sucrose, 9.76 g of glucose and 9.94 g of fructose to 100 ml of semi-skimmed milk).	It was identified that anthocyanins (143 mg) present in blueberry juice have memory benefits in children aged 8 to 10 years, however, little evidence in attention, visuospatial, working memory were observed.

Table 3.
Recent research in humans and animal models related to supplementation with berries.

considered the main mechanism of action [106], since oxidative stress has been proposed as an important contributor to anxiety generation [79].

5.2 Depression

Depression is the most prevalent psychiatric disorder; according to the World Health Organization, it affects 300 million people worldwide [97]. Depressive disorders are characterized by the presence of a sad and irritable mood accompanied by somatic and cognitive changes that negatively impact everyday life function [97] and result in high financial costs [111]. A great variety of drugs exist for its treatment [112], in which therapeutic effects are driven by actions on diverse neurotransmission systems (serotonergic, dopaminergic, and noradrenergic), exerting long-term changes which can restore neuronal function, for example, restoration of basal levels of neurotransmitters mainly serotonin, increase in neurotrophic factors (brain-derived neurotrophic factor and nerve growth factor) that can indirectly modify neuronal microarchitecture, reduction of oxidative stress, as well as neuroinflammation processes in structures related to the pathophysiology of depression which can impact at the affective level exerting favorable effects on the quality of life of the subjects. These drugs include tricyclic antidepressants (i.e., imipramine), selective serotonin recapture inhibitors (i.e., fluoxetine), monoamine oxidase inhibitors (phenelzine), and dual antidrepressant drugs (venlafaxine), among others [113]. Most of these drugs have a late onset and are often accompanied by side effects when taken for prolonged periods. This has encouraged a search for new substances with potential antidepressant effects and, most importantly, the use of possible natural alternatives.

An association between the role the hippocampus and the etiology of depression has been suggested, given that a reduction in hippocampal neurogenesis has been observed in depressed patients with respect to the non-depressed control group, which is accompanied by a decrease in the hippocampal volume [114]. In this sense, antidepressants such as fluoxetine have been shown to ameliorate neurogenesis in the hippocampus [115].

At the preclinical level, the administration of *Aronia melanocarpa* juice showed a decrease in total immobility time in the forced swimming test [107], similar to animals treated with imipramine. In addition, the study was supplemented with in vitro testing, where inhibition of the enzyme monoamine oxidase was observed, both in its A form and to a lesser extent in its B form [104]. MAO-A and MAO-B inhibitors are used clinically for the treatment of psychiatric and neurological disorders, respectively [116]. This activity has been proposed as another mechanism for the action of berries in mental disorders, as it is related to increased levels of serotonin, dopamine, and noradrenaline.

In addition, human studies related to blueberry and red berry supplementation have shown that a higher intake of these foods is associated with a lower risk of depression [85, 86]. Similarly, studies in mice have shown similar effects with the consumption of red berries, observing a reduction in depressive-like behaviors [87, 88] (**Table 3**).

5.3 Alzheimer's disease

Alzheimer's disease (AD) is a neurodegenerative disorder characterized by progressive memory loss, as well as cognitive decline [117] in which prevalence augments with age [118]. The neuropathologic changes underlying AD include senile plaques formed by the peptide β-amyloid and neurofibrillary tangles composed of hyperphosphorylated Tau protein that promotes synaptic dysfunction and neuronal death early and consistently [119].

Oxidative stress has been associated with the onset and progression of AD [120]. This is supported by the high vulnerability of neurons to reactive oxygen species (ROS) [121]. Oxidative stress can induce damage to membrane lipids, changes in glial and neuronal function, structural damage to DNA, synaptic dysfunction, and apoptosis [122].

Several studies have demonstrated the potential protective effect of blackberry fruits (*Rubus L.* subgenus *Rubus Watson*), in the prevention of age-related neurodegenerative disorders [123], specifically with PD. Berry fruits such as blackberry, black raspberry, blueberry, and strawberry are good sources of phytochemicals that provide protection against neurological disorders [93].

Extracts of black currant have been shown to inhibit the formation and spread of β-amyloid [124] and ROS fibrils. Supplementation of blackberry in in vitro studies has been reported to exhibit potent anti-inflammatory and antiproliferative properties [125, 126]; also, the consumption of blueberries is related to neuronal augment in the hippocampus [5].

Recently a neuroprotective effect of anthocyanins has been observed in a model of AD induced by streptozotocin that resulted in a cognitive deficit (in short-term memory and spatial memory), as well as dysfunction in the activity of the enzyme acetylcholinesterase, while inducing lipid peroxidation and a decrease in antioxidant enzymes in the cerebral cortex [127]. These alterations were attenuated in the group administered with anthocyanins. Similarly, it has been observed that blueberry powder (*Vaccinium* sp.) supplementation in patients with Alzheimer's disease and cognitive decline reduces the self-reported inefficiencies in daily functioning [90] (**Table 3**).

5.4 Parkinson's disease

Parkinson's disease (PD) is characterized by tremors, stiffness, and akinesia. It is caused by the progressive degeneration of dopaminergic neurons in the substantia nigra and the presence of Lewy bodies. Many Parkinson's risks and preventive factors have been investigated. The onset of this disorder has been associated with exposure to certain pesticides and heavy metals [128], tobacco consumption [129], and coffee consumption [130], among other environmental factors. While current treatments have shown effectiveness in early management of the motor symptoms of the disease [131] and both surgery and deep brain stimulation are useful, PD is currently not yet curable [132]. A diet enriched in phenolic compounds has been shown to have some efficacy in relieving Parkinson's symptoms [133]. Most of the studies related to fruit consumption and disease focus on supplementation with blueberries, strawberries, black currant, and grapes, due to their powerful antioxidant effects related to their high content of polyphenols and anthocyanins [134].

Cell models have reinforced studies of neurodegenerative disorders, recently demonstrating that anthocyanins from grape seed, blueberry, and mulberry enhance mitochondrial function [135] and suppressed dopaminergic cell death caused by rotenone (insecticide and pesticide) in mitochondrial respiration. This has suggested that anthocyanins may alleviate neurodegeneration in PD by improving mitochondrial function. In addition, polyphenols are able to ameliorate inflammatory responses associated with glial activation [136]. Phenolic compounds are known for their ability to eliminate reactive oxygen species (ROS) due to their antioxidant action; however, since their concentrations in the brain are lower than those of endogenous antioxidants, it has begun to be seen that they also exert their neuroprotective effects through additional mechanisms [137, 138], highlighting the inhibition of MAO, in its two forms, A and B [77, 104]. At the preclinical level, one of the most widely used models in PD research is the administration of 1-methyl-4-phenyl-1,2,3,6-tetrahydropyridine (MPTP), a neurotoxin that causes a severe Parkinson's-like syndrome in humans, monkeys, and mice [139–142]. It has been observed that daily administration of resveratrol (red wine polyphenol) in male mice C57BL/6 prevented a decrease in striatal dopamine and maintained striatal tyrosine hydroxylase levels. In addition, mice that received resveratrol as pretreatment showed a greater number of immunopositive tyrosine hydroxylase neurons, indicating the protective role of resveratrol over nigral neurons [143]. In the same disease model, it was observed that blueberry extract attenuated behavioral impairment (motor coordination) as well as decreased levels of malondialdehyde in the brains of mice [92]. These data reveal the ability of resveratrol and polyphenols present in blueberry extract to counteract the toxic effects of MPTP administration and in the near future may be used as a complementary neuroprotective therapy (**Table 3**). Current PD therapies act by controlling the disease's symptoms, but do not slow the underlying neurodegeneration in the brains of PD in patients [135]; this is an opportunity to use functional foods as adjuvant therapy in the presence of disease.

5.5 Human cognition

Polyphenols present in berries have also been associated with cognitive amelioration and neuronal function, as is the case with grape juice, which in both young [144] and older adults [145] ameliorate neurocognitive functions of memory, attention, and calmness, compared to the placebo group. In this same regard, in mothers (40–50 years) of preadolescent children, an association of grape juice consumption has been observed (≥30 h/week 355 ml, during 12 weeks) with subtle augment in immediate spatial memory and safer driving behavior in a virtual simulator [146]. At the same time, it was found that, in a double-blind crossover design of children (7 and 10 years old), supplementation of 15 or 30 g freeze-dried wild blueberry powder significantly ameliorates word acquisition and recognition, as well as the ability to overcome the effects of response interference [147].

In a pilot study in healthy young adults in both genders (18–35 years old), it has been observed that the acute administration of black currant juice (500 mg/day of polyphenols, supplemented only 1 day per week, during 31 days) exerts an anxiolytic-like effect, as well as ameliorates alertness, less fatigue, and reaction speed [94].

In a randomized, double-blind placebo-controlled trial, dietary blueberry of 24 g/day for 3 months raised the cognition in tests of executive function in adults between 60 and 75 years old of both sexes by increasing accuracy during task switching and reduced repetition errors during word-list recall [148]. The positive effects on cognition have been related to activation of the prefrontal cortex using functional magnetic resonance imaging [149]; therefore, the administration of blueberry to have the same effects on these tasks could be exercising greater activation of this structure to raise cognition. Another study found that daily consumption of 6 and 9 ml/kg for 12 weeks of blueberry (*Vaccinium angustifolium* Aiton) juice exerted neurocognitive benefits measured by California Verbal Learning Test-II (CVLT) augmented associate learning and word-list recall in older adults of both sexes who had experienced age-related memory decline [145]. Similarly, randomized controlled trial has shown that dietary berry juice (200 ml/day) for 12 weeks ameliorate memory and cognition in adults (70–80 years old) with cognitive impairment measured using a battery Rey Auditory Verbal Learning Test (RAVLT) [150].

Furthermore, a randomized, double-blind, placebo-controlled study showed that the daily administration of two capsules (10o mg) of a purified extract of blueberry (wild blueberry extract) for 3 months raised episodic and working memory in older adults of both sexes [151]. Additionally, a randomized, single-blind, parallel group design showed that the acute consumption of 200 ml of wild blueberry drink (253 mg anthocyanins) in healthy children aged 7–10 years significantly enhanced the memory and attentional aspects of executive function with respect to the placebo group 2 h after consumption; therefore, the consumption of the wild blueberry drink during the critical period of development (as is the case of childhood) could provide acute cognitive benefits [152]. Therefore, a double-blind, counterbalanced, crossover intervention study showed that acute supplementation with haskap berry extract "*Lonicera caerulea* L." (200 and 400 mg anthocyanins) raised the episodic memory and exerts benefits in cognitive performance following a single acute dose in older adults compared to placebo [153].

These findings support that the consumption of berries produces beneficial effects on cognition in humans, which are probably related to the effects of the berries on the nervous system. For example, blueberry diets are associated with enhanced working memory which is accompanied by an increase in the neurogenesis of the hippocampus [17]. A randomized, controlled, double-blind, crossover studio showed that the administration of 766 mg total blueberry polyphenols in healthy young men reduced neutrophil NADPH oxidase activity at 1, 2, 4, and 6 h after consumption [154]. In this sense, NADPH oxidase has been shown to play an important role in oxidative stress induction in the brain [155], because it uses oxygen and NADPH to generate superoxide [156]. Therefore, the administration of blueberry could be generating a reduction of superoxide and indirectly preventing oxidative stress events a long term. The mechanisms by which flavonoids and polyphenols exert these actions on cognitive performance are still being studied, including evidence suggesting that they can increase brain blood flow, as well as modulate the activation state of neuronal receptors, signaling proteins, and gene expression [157].

6. Berry side or toxicity effect

According to our knowledge, there are some reports relating berry consumption in humans with side effects or toxicity. Data of toxicity in vivo was reported in 1997, in a study of the relation between flavonoid intake and subsequent cancer risk in 9959 Finnish men and women, aged 15–99 years and who are initially cancer free. Food consumption and dietary history method calculated the consumption of lingonberries, blueberries, black currants, raspberries, and gooseberries. People with higher consumption of berries were found to have a high risk of lung cancer. Apparently, the phenolic compounds produce toxicity proliferating cancer cells, but are not toxic in healthy cells [49].

Another study of 5-weeks-old Swiss Webster male mice, supplemented with lyophilized nightshade berries (*Solanum dulcamara*, 8 g/kg) with two different stages of maturity, showed that immature fruit supplementation produced gastrointestinal lesions; however, this condition was not observed in mice administered with mature lyophilized fruit. The authors concluded that these effects were attributed to the presence of saponin in the immature fruit [158]. In 2015, the first toxicity report by *Solanum dulcamara* was reported in a dog puppy (Labrador Retriever); the toxicity was attributed to steroidal glycoalkaloid solanine. After causing vomiting to the dog, dried stems and immature berries were observed, and gastric contents were evaluated by a local botanist identifying *Solanum dulcamara* intake, concluding that dog poisoning was due to the consumption of this fruit [159].

Another report was in 2009, when dozens of dead cedar waxwings in Thomas County, Georgia, USA, were found. In this case report, after evaluating five birds, the investigation group observed pulmonary, mediastinal, and tracheal hemorrhages and also found berries (*Nandina domestica* Thunb.) intact and partly digested into the gastrointestinal tracts. Due to their voracious feeding behavior, these birds ingested toxic doses of *N. domestica* and at the same time high concentrations of cyanide present in fruit berry [160]. It is important to note that *S. dulcamara* and *N. domestica* species are found wildly and are not consumed by humans.

Regarding berries supplementation and synergy, it is recently reported that gallic acid, quercetin, ellagic acid, and cyanidin have a market antioxidant activity [161, 162], due to the synergistic effects between the numbers of aromatic ring mixtures. In addition, polyphenols present in berries can interact between them, improve their antioxidant properties, and, therefore, increase human's health benefits [162]. According to our knowledge, no studies were found related with pharmacological interactions and berry supplementation. It is necessary to carry out studies involving pharmacological molecules, berries' activities, and their phenolic compounds in order to generate new therapies and identify the existence of side or toxic effects.

7. Final comments

According to the research reported in this chapter, the supplementation of berries and their bioactive compounds as flavonoids, polyphenols, and anthocyanin suggests a potential health benefit for human nutrition.

The objective of this research is to contribute with knowledge to the development of new strategies for the treatment of diseases such as anxiety, depression, AD, and PD, which includes natural products, particularly berry fruits that work as preventive or coadjuvant therapy in the treatment of these diseases.

A further evaluation of fruits berry supplementation in neural processes is required, as well as the identification of the effect of each particular bioactive compound on psychiatric and neurological disorders. More studies will be necessary to identify the mechanisms of action of this substance. It is also important to understand the scope in other neural processes and their application, effectiveness, synergy, pharmacological interaction, and side or toxic effects at clinical and preclinical levels of studies.

8. Conclusions

The present chapter evidenced a number of investigations in vivo related with the use of different berry fruit supplement doses, not only in humans but also in animal models. These results suggest the potential health effect of berries due to bioactive compounds mainly flavonoids, polyphenols, and anthocyanins, used commonly for its antioxidant capacity. According to our knowledge, the cases reported in the literature by animal toxicity are related with the consumption of wild berries. In humans the relationship between phenol compound consumption and lung cancer has been reported; however, there is no evidence of side or toxic effects related with berry supplementation or their bioactive compounds, and pharmacological interaction related to their consumption due to no dietary intervention studies has been reported.

In addition, berry consumption has shown to be effective in a number of cardiovascular and metabolic diseases, and also recent investigations are proposed for the management of berry fruit supplementation as neuroprotector and the reduction of symptoms in diseases such as anxiety, depression, AD, and PD, among others. The use of this biological berry compounds might promote an alternative for prevention and give excellent opportunities for human nutrition as a functional food and nutraceutical. Future research in this field is necessary, in order to clarify and support the evidence of the effects of flavonoids, polyphenols, and anthocyanins at the brain level, as well as their potential direct and indirect mechanisms of action.

Acknowledgements

The authors gratefully acknowledge the financial support from CONACyT (Scholarship no. 592714, 628503, 297410, 713495).

Conflict of interest

The authors declare no conflict of interest.

Author details

Fernández-Demeneghi Rafael[1], Vargas-Moreno Isidro[1], Acosta-Mesa Héctor-Gabriel[2], Puga-Olguín Abraham[1], Campos-Uscanga Yolanda[3], Romo-González Tania[4], Guzmán-Gerónimo Rosa-Isela[5], Patraca-Camacho Lorena[1] and Herrera-Meza Socorro[6*]

1 Institute of Neuroethology, University of Veracruz, Xalapa, Veracruz, Mexico

2 Artificial Intelligence Research Center, University of Veracruz, Xalapa, Veracruz, Mexico

3 Institute of Public Health, University of Veracruz, Xalapa, Veracruz, Mexico

4 Institute of Biological Research, University of Veracruz, Xalapa, Veracruz, Mexico

5 Basic Sciences Institute, University of Veracruz, Xalapa, Veracruz, Mexico

6 Institute of Psychological Research, University of Veracruz, Xalapa, Veracruz, Mexico

*Address all correspondence to: soherrera@uv.mx

References

[1] Nile S, Park S. Edible berries: Bioactive components and their effect on human health. Nutrition. 2014;**30**:134-144. DOI: 10.1016/j.nut.2013.04.007

[2] Andres-Lacueva C, Shukitt-Hale B, Galli R, Jauregui O, Lamuela-Raventos R, Joseph J. Anthocyanins in aged blueberry-fed rats are found centrally and may enhance memory. Nutritional Neuroscience. 2005;**8**:111-120. DOI: 10.1080/10284150500078117

[3] Talavéra S, Felgines C, Texier O, Besson C, Gil-Izquierdo A, Lamaison J, et al. Anthocyanin metabolism in rats and their distribution to digestive area, kidney, and brain. Journal of Agricultural and Food Chemistry. 2005;**53**:3902-3908. DOI: 10.1021/jf050145v

[4] Fernández-Demeneghi R, Rodríguez-Landa J, Guzmán-Gerónimo R, Acosta-Mesa H, Meza-Alvarado E, Vargas-Moreno I, et al. Effect of blackberry juice (*Rubus fruticosus* L.) on anxiety-like behaviour in Wistar rats. International Journal of Food Sciences and Nutrition. 2019;**70**:1-12. DOI: 10.1080/09637486.2019.1580680

[5] Casadesus G, Shukitt-Hale B, Stellwagen H, Zhu X, Lee H, Smith M, et al. Modulation of hippocampal plasticity and cognitive behavior by short-term blueberry supplementation in aged rats. Nutritional Neuroscience. 2004;7:309-316. DOI: 10.1080/10284150400020482

[6] Martirosyan D, Singh J. A new definition of functional food by FFC: What makes a new definition unique. FFHD. 2015;**5**:209-223. DOI: 10.31989/ffhd.v5i6.183

[7] Santini A, Tenore G, Novellino E. Nutraceuticals: A paradigm of proactive medicine. European Journal of Pharmaceutical Sciences. 2017;**96**:53-61. DOI: 10.1016/j.ejps.2016.09.003

[8] McDougall G, Stewart D. The inhibitory effects of berry polyphenols on digestive enzymes. BioFactors. 2006;**27**:189-195. DOI: 10.1002/biof.5520230403

[9] Chaves V, Boff L, Vizzotto M, Calvete E, Reginatto F, Simões C. Berries grown in Brazil: Anthocyanin profiles and biological properties. Journal of Science and Food Agriculture. 2018;**98**:4331-4338. DOI: 10.1002/jsfa.8959

[10] Lau F, Bielinski D, Joseph J. Inhibitory effects of blueberry extract on the production of inflammatory mediators in lipopolysaccharide-activated BV2 microglia. Journal of Neuroscience Research. 2007;**85**:1010-1017. DOI: 10.1002/jnr.21205

[11] Williamson G. Possible effects of dietary polyphenols on sugar absorption and digestion. Molecular Nutrition & Food Research. 2013;**57**:48-57. DOI: 10.1002/mnfr.20120051117

[12] Krishna G, Ying Z, Gomez-Pinilla F. Blueberry supplementation mitigates altered brain plasticity and behaviour after traumatic brain injury in rats. Molecular Nutrition & Food Research. 2019;**63**:1-8. DOI: 10.1002/mnfr.201801055

[13] Kalt W, Blumberg J, McDonald J, Vinqvist-Tymchuk M, Fillmore S, Graf B, et al. Identification of anthocyanins in the liver, eye, and brain of blueberry-fed pigs. Journal of Agricultural and Food Chemistry. 2008;**56**:705-712. DOI: 10.1021/jf071998l

[14] Bowen-Forbes C, Zhang Y, Muraleedharan N. Anthocyanin content, antioxidant, anti-inflammatory

and anticancer properties of blackberry and raspeberry fruits. Journal of Food Composition and Analysis. 2010;**23**: 554-560. DOI: 10.1016/j.jfca.2009.08.012

[15] Hampto S, Isherwood C, Kirkpatrick V, Lynne-Smith A, Griffin B. The influence of alcohol consumed with a meal on endothelial function in healthy individuals. Journal of Human Nutrition and Dietetics. 2010;**23**: 120-125. DOI: 10.1111/j.1365-277X.2009.01021.x

[16] Zhao M, Liu X, Luo Y, Guo H, Hu X, Chen F. Evaluation of protective effect of freeze-dried strawberry, grape, and blueberry powder on acrylamide toxicity in mice. Journal of Food Science. 2015;**80**:869-874. DOI: 10.1111/1750-3841.12815

[17] Shukitt-Hale B, Bielinski D, Lau F, Willis L, Carey A, Joseph J. The beneficial effects of berries on cognition, motor behaviour and neuronal function in ageing. British Journal of Nutrition. 2015;**114**:1542-1549. DOI: 10.1017/S0007114515003451

[18] Dohadwala M, Holbrook M, Hamburg N, Shenouda S, Chun W, Titas M, et al. Effects of cranberry juice consumption on vascular function in patients with coronary artery disease. The American Journal of Clinical Nutrition. 2011;**93**:934-940. DOI: 10.3945/ajcn.110.004242

[19] Barros D, Amaral B, Izquierdo I, Geracitano L, Raseira M, Henriques A, et al. Behavioral and genoprotective effects of Vaccinium berries intake in mice. Pharmacology Biochemistry & Behavior. 2006;**84**:229-234. DOI: 10.1016/j.pbb.2006.05.001

[20] Miller M, Shukitt-Hale B. Berry fruit enhances beneficial signaling in the brain. Journal of Agricultural and Food Chemistry. 2012;**60**:5709-5715. DOI: 10.1021/jf2036033

[21] Baby B, Antony P, Vijayan R. Antioxidant and anticancer properties of berries. Critical Reviews in Food Science and Nutrition. 2018;**58**:2491-2507. DOI: 10.1080/10408398.2017.1329198

[22] Diaconeasa Z, Leopold L, Rugină D, Ayvaz H, Socaciu C. Antiproliferative and antioxidant properties of anthocyanin rich extracts from blueberry and blackcurrant juice. International Journal of Molecular Sciences. 2015;**16**:2352-2365. DOI: 10.3390/ijms16022352

[23] Pantelidis G, Vasilakakis M, ManganarisG,DiamantidisG.Antioxidant capacity, phenol, anthocyanin and ascorbic acid contents in raspberries, blackberries, red currants, gooseberries and cornelian cherries. Food Chemistry. 2007;**102**:777-783. DOI: 10.1016/j.foodchem.2006.06.021

[24] Lorenzo J, Pateiro M, Domínguez R, Barba F, Putnik P, Kovačević D, et al. Berries extracts as natural antioxidants in meat products: A review. Food Research International. 2018;**106**:1095-1104. DOI: 10.1016/j.foodres.2017.12.005

[25] Wang S, Lin H. Antioxidant activity in fruits and leaves of blackberry, raspberry, and strawberry varies with cultivar and developmental stage. Journal of Agricultural and Food Chemistry. 2010;**48**:140-146. DOI: 10.1021/jf9908345I

[26] Lee S, Vance T, Nam T, Kim D, Koo S, Chun O. Contribution of anthocyanin composition to total antioxidant capacity of berries. Plant Food for Human Nutrition. 2015;**70**:427-432. DOI: 10.1007/s11130-015-0514-5

[27] Rabassa M, Trespalacios M, Urpi-Sarda M, Llorach R, Tulípani S, Zamora-Ros M, et al. Polifenoles como antioxidantes. In: Álvarez E, González A, De la Rosa L, Ayala J, editors. Antioxidantes en Alimentos y Salud.

1st ed. Ameditores: Cdmx; 2012. pp. 155-200

[28] Estrada-Reyes R, Ubaldo-Suárez D, Araujo-Escalona A. Los flavonoides y el sistema nervioso central. Salud Mental. 2012;**35**:375-384

[29] Ono K, Yoshiike Y, Takashima A, Hasegawa K, Naiki H, Yamada M. Potent anti-amyloidogenic and fibril-destabilizing effects of polyphenols in vitro: Implications for the prevention and therapeutics of Alzheimer's disease. Journal of Neurochemistry. 2003;**87**: 172-181. DOI: 10.1046/j.1471-4159. 2003.01976.x

[30] Sellappan S, Akoh C, Krewer G. Phenolic compounds and antioxidant capacity of Georgia-grown blueberries and blackberries. Journal of Agricultural and Food Chemistry. 2012;**50**:2432-2438. DOI: 10.1021/jf011097r

[31] Vignes M, Maurice T, Lanté F, Nedjar M, Thethi K, Guiramand J, et al. Anxiolytic properties of green tea polyphenol (−)-epigallocatechin gallate (EGCG). Brain Research. 2006;**1110**:102-115. DOI: 10.1016/j. brainres.2006.06.062

[32] De la Peña J, Kim C, Lee H, Yoon S, Kim H, Hong E, et al. Luteolin mediates the antidepressant-like effects of Cirsium japonicum in mice, possibly through modulation of the GABAA receptor. Archives of Pharmacal Research. 2014;**37**:263-269. DOI: 10.1007/s12272-013-0229-9

[33] Johnston G. GABAA receptor channel pharmacology. Current Pharmaceutical Design. 2005;**11**:1867-1885. DOI: 10.2174/1381612054021024

[34] Hanrahan J, Chebib M, Johnston G. Interactions of flavonoids with ionotropic GABA receptors. Advances in Pharmacology. 2015;**72**:189-200. DOI: 10.1016/bs.apha.2014.10.007

[35] Youdim K, Shukitt-Hale B, Joseph J. Flavonoids and the brain: Interactions at the blood–brain barrier and their physiological effects on the central nervous system. Free Radical Biology and Medicine. 2004;**37**:1683-1693. DOI: 10.1016/j. freeradbiomed.2004.08.002

[36] Jäger A, Saaby L. Flavonoids and the CNS. Molecules. 2011;**16**:1471-1485. DOI: 10.3390/molecules160214/1

[37] Cho S, Han D, Yang H, Jeon Y, Lee C, Jin Y, et al. Phlorotannins of the edible brown seaweed Ecklonia cava Kjellman induce sleep via positive allosteric modulation of gamma-aminobutyric acid type A–benzodiazepine receptor: A novel neurological activity of seaweed polyphenols. Food Chemistry. 2012;**132**:1133-1142. DOI: 10.1016/j. foodchem.2011.08.040

[38] Perez-Vizcaino F, Duarte J, Jimenez R, Santos-Buelga C, Osuna A. Antihypertensive effects of the flavonoid quercetin. Pharmacological Reports. 2009;**61**:7-75. DOI: 10.1016/S1734-1140(09)70008-8

[39] Quiñones M, Miguel M, Aleixandre A. Los polifenoles, compuestos de origen natural con efectos saludables sobre el sistema cardiovascular. Nutrición Hospitalaria. 2012;**77**:76-89. DOI: 10.3305/ nh.2012.27.1.5418

[40] Ferraro F, Balota D, Connor L. Implicit memory and the formation of new associations in nondemented Parkinson's disease individuals and individuals with senile dementia of the Alzheimer type: A serial reaction time (SRT) investigation. Brain and Cognition. 1993;**21**:163-180. DOI: 10.1006/brcg.1993.1013

[41] Narayana K, Reddy M, Chaluvadi M, Krishna D. Bioflavonoids classification, pharmacological, biochemical effects and therapeutic potential. Indian Journal of Pharmacology. 2001;**33**:2-16

[42] Kujumgiev A, Tsvetkova I, Serkedjieva Y, Bankova V, Christov R, Popov S. Antibacterial, antifungal and antiviral activity of propolis of different geographic origin. Journal of Ethnopharmacology. 1999;**64**:235-240. DOI: 10.1016/s0378-8741(98)00131-7

[43] De Lira Mota K, Días G, Pinto M, Luiz-Ferreira Â, Monteiro A, Hiruma-Lima C, et al. Flavonoids with gastroprotective activity. Molecules. 2009;**14**:979-1012. DOI: 10.3390/molecules14030979

[44] Nishino H, Ono T, Muramoto K, Fukuda M, Sasaki K. Neuronal activity in the ventral tegmental area (VTA) during motivated bar press feeding in the monkey. Brain Research. 1987;**413**:302-313. DOI: 10.1016/0006-8993(87)91021-3

[45] Bahadoran Z, Mirmiran P, Azizi F. Dietary polyphenols as potential nutraceuticals in management of diabetes: A review. Journal of Diabetes and Metabolic Disorders. 2013;**12**:1-9. DOI: 10.1186/2251-6581-12-43

[46] Guerrero-Legarreta I, López-Hernández E, Armenta-López R, García-Barrientos R. Pigmentos. In: Lópéz-Vallesteros G, editor. Química de los Alimentos. 5th ed. Mexico: Pearson Educación; 2013. pp. 379-428

[47] Strack D, Wray V, Metzger J, Grosse W. Two anthocyanins acylated with gallic acid from the leaves of *Victoria amazonica*. Phytochemistry. 1992;**31**:989-991. DOI: 10.1016/0031-9422(92)80054-I

[48] Manach C, Scalbert A, Morand C, Rémésy C, Jiménez L. Polyphenols: Food sources and bioavailability. The American Journal of Clinical Nutrition. 2004;**79**:727-747. DOI: 10.1093/ajcn/79.5.727

[49] Knekt P, Järvinen R, Seppänen R, Heliövaara M, Teppo L, Pukkala E, et al. Dietary flavonoids and the risk of lung cancer and other malignant neoplasms. American Journal of Epidemiology. 1997;**146**:223-230. DOI: 10.1093/oxfordjournals.aje.a009257

[50] Arai Y, Watanabe S, Kimira M, Shimoi K, Mochizuki R, Kinae N. Dietary intakes of flavonols, flavones and isoflavones by Japanese women and the inverse correlation between quercetin intake and plasma LDL cholesterol concentration. The Journal of Nutrition. 2000;**130**:2243-2250. DOI: 10.1093/jn/130.9.2243

[51] Izzo A, Carlo G, Mascolo N, Capasso F, Autore G. Antiulcer effect of flavonoids. Role of endogenous PAF. Phytotherapy Research. 1994;**8**:179-181. DOI: 10.1002/ptr.2650080313

[52] Yilmaz I, Hatipoglu H, Taslidere E, Karaaslan M. Comparing the regenerative effects of Silymarin and Apricot on liver regeneration after partial hepatectomy in rats. Biomedical Research. 2018;**26**:1465-1473. DOI: 10.4066/biomedicalresearch.29-17-2142

[53] Matsuzaki K, Miyazaki K, Sakai S, Yawo H, Nakata N, Moriguchi S, et al. Nobiletin, a citrus flavonoid with neurotrophic action, augments protein kinase A-mediated phosphorylation of the AMPA receptor subunit, GluR1, and the postsynaptic receptor response to glutamate in murine hippocampus. European Journal of Pharmacology. 2008;**578**:194-200. DOI: 10.1016/j.ejphar.2007.09.028

[54] Zelus C, Fox A, Calciano A, Faridian B, Nogaj L, Moffet D. Myricetin inhibits islet amyloid polypeptide (IAPP) aggregation and rescues living mammalian cells from IAPP toxicity. Open Biochemistry Journal. 2012;**6**:66. DOI: 10.2174/1874091X01206010066

[55] Bournival J, Plouffe M, Renaud J, Provencher C, Quercetin MM. Sesamin protect dopaminergic cells from MPP.

Oxidative Medicine and Cellular Longevity. 2012;**2012**:921-941. DOI: 10.1155/2012/921941

[56] Machado D, Bettio L, Cunha M, Santos A, Pizzolatti M, Brighente I, et al. Antidepressant-like effect of rutin isolated from the ethanolic extract from *Schinus molle* L. in mice: Evidence for the involvement of the serotonergic and noradrenergic systems. European Journal of Pharmacology. 2008;**587**:163-168. DOI: 10.1016/j.ejphar.2008.03.021

[57] German-Ponciano L, Dutra B, Miranda L, Dos Santos K, Da Silva S, Cueto-Escobedo J, Lima-Maximino M, Rodríguez-Landa J, Maximino C. Chrysin, but not the flavone backbone, decreases anxiety-like behavior in animal tests. BioRxiv. DOI: 10.1101/575514

[58] Melo M, Pina F, Andary C. Anthocyanins: Nature's glamorous palette. In: Bechtold T, Mussak R, editors. Handbook of Natural Colorants. Chichester: Wiley; 2009. pp. 134-150

[59] Yoshida K, Mori M, Kondo T. Blue flower color development by anthocyanins: From chemical structure to cell physiology. Natural Product Reports. 2009;**26**:884-915. DOI: 10.1039-b800165k

[60] Castaneda-Ovando A, de Lourdes Pacheco-Hernández M, Páez-Hernández M, Rodríguez J, Galán-Vidal C. Chemical studies of anthocyanins: A review. Food Chemistry. 2009;**113**:859-871. DOI: 10.1016/j.foodchem.2008.09.001

[61] Collado J. Identificación de los polifenoles en zumos de frutas rojas [thesis]. Colombia–Cartagena: Universidad Politécnica de Cartagena; 2011

[62] Kong J, Chia L, Goh N, Chia T, Brouillard R. Analysis and biological activities of anthocyanins. Phytochemistry. 2003;**64**:923-933. DOI: 10.1016/S0031-9422(03)00438-2

[63] Kuskoski E, Asuero A, García-Parilla M, Troncoso A, Fett R. Actividad antioxidante de pigmentos antociánicos. Food Science and Technology. 2004;**24**:691-693. DOI: 10.1590/S0101-20612004000400036

[64] Chen P, Chu S, Chiou H, Kuo W, Chiang C, Hsieh Y. Mulberry anthocyanins, cyanidin 3-rutinoside and cyanidin 3-glucoside, exhibited an inhibitory effect on the migration and invasion of a human lung cancer cell line. Cancer Letters. 2006;**235**:248-259. DOI: 10.1016/j.canlet.2005.04.033

[65] Ding M, Feng R, Wang S, Bowman L, Lu Y, Qian Y, et al. Cyanidin-3-glucoside, a natural product derived from blackberry, exhibits chemopreventive and chemotherapeutic activity. Journal of Biological Chemistry. 2016;**281**:17359-17368. DOI: 10.1074/jbc.M600861200

[66] Cuevas-Rodriguez E, Yousef G, Garcia-Saucedo P, Lopez-Medina J, Paredes-López O, Lila M. Characterization of anthocyanins and proanthocyanidins in wild and domesticated Mexican blackberries (Rubus spp.). Journal of Agricultural and Food Chemistry. 2010;**58**:7458-7464. DOI: 10.1021/jf101485r

[67] Garzón G. Las antocianinas como colorantes naturales y compuestos bioactivos: revisión. Acta Biológica Colombiana. 2008;**13**:27-36

[68] Kirakosyan A, Seymour E, Wolforth J, McNish R, Kaufman P, Bolling S. Tissue bioavailability of anthocyanins from whole tart cherry in healthy rats. Food Chemistry. 2015;**171**:26-31. DOI: 10.1016/j.foodchem.2014.08.114

[69] Santos-Buelga C, Mateus N, De Freitas V. Anthocyanins. Plant pigments and beyond. Journal of Agricultural and

Food Chemistry. 2014;**62**:6879-6884. DOI: 10.1021/jf501950s

[70] Wang D, Wei X, Yan X, Jin T, Ling W. Protocatechuic acid, a metabolite of anthocyanins, inhibits monocyte adhesion and reduces atherosclerosis in apolipoprotein E-deficient mice. Journal of Agricultural and Food Chemistry. 2010;**58**:12722-12728. DOI: 10.1021/jf103427j

[71] Wallace T. Anthocyanins in cardiovascular disease. Advances in Nutrition. 2011;**2**:1-7. DOI: 10.3945/an.110.000042

[72] Kamei H, Kojima T, Hasegawa M, Koide T, Umeda T, Yukawa T, et al. Suppression of tumor cell growth by anthocyanins in vitro. Cancer Investigation. 1995;**13**:590-594. DOI: 10.3109/07357909509024927

[73] Hidalgo M, Martin-Santamaria S, Recio I, Sanchez-Moreno C, de Pascual-Teresa B, Rimbach G, et al. Potential anti-inflammatory, anti-adhesive, anti/estrogenic, and angiotensin-converting enzyme inhibitory activities of anthocyanins and their gut metabolites. Genes & Nutrition. 2012;**7**:295-306. DOI: 10.1007_s12263-011-0263-5

[74] Rojo L, Ribnicky D, Logendra S, Poulev A, Rojas-Silva P, Kuhn P, et al. In vitro and in vivo anti-diabetic effects of anthocyanins from Maqui Berry (*Aristotelia chilensis*). Food Chemistry. 2012;**131**:387-396. DOI: 10.1016/j.foodchem.2011.08.066

[75] Zafra-Stone S, Yasmin T, Bagchi M, Chatterjee A, Vinson J, Bagchi D. Berry anthocyanins as novel antioxidants in human health and disease prevention. Molecular Nutrition & Food Research. 2007;**51**:675-683. DOI: 10.1002/mnfr.200700002

[76] Pribis P, Shukitt-Hale B. Cognition: The new frontier for nuts and berries. The American Journal of Clinical Nutrition. 2014;**100**:347S-352S. DOI: 10.3945/ajcn.113.071506

[77] Dreiseitel A, Korte G, Schreier P, Oehme A, Locher S, Domani M, et al. Berry anthocyanins and their aglycons inhibit monoamine oxidases A and B. Pharmacological Research. 2009;**59**:306-311. DOI: 10.1016/j.phrs.2009.01.014

[78] Joseph J, Shukitt-Hale B, Brewer G, Weikel K, Kalt W, Fisher D. Differential protection among fractionated blueberry polyphenolic families against DA-, Aβ42-and LPS-induced decrements in Ca^{2+} buffering in primary hippocampal cells. Journal of Agricultural and Food Chemistry. 2010;**58**:8196-8204. DOI: 10.1021/jf100144y

[79] Bouayed J, Hoffmann L, Bohn T. Total phenolics, flavonoids, anthocyanins and antioxidant activity following simulated gastro-intestinal digestion and dialysis of apple varieties: Bioaccessibility and potential uptake. Food Chemistry. 2011;**128**:14-21. DOI: 10.1016/j.foodchem.2011.02.052

[80] Wang S, Jiao H. Scavenging capacity of berry crops on superoxide radicals, hydrogen peroxide, hydroxyl radicals, and singlet oxygen. Journal of Agricultural and Food Chemistry. 2000;**48**:5677-5684. DOI: 10.1021/jf000766i

[81] Wang Y, Lin H. Antioxidant activity in fruits and leaves of blackberry, raspberry, and strawberry varies with cultivar and developmental stage. Journal of Agricultural and Food Chemistry. 2000;**48**:40-146. DOI: 10.1021/jf9908345

[82] Kim H, Ju M, Shim J, Kim M, Lee S, Huh Y, et al. Mulberry fruit protects dopaminergic neurons in toxin-induced Parkinson's disease models. British Journal of Nutrition. 2010;**104**:8-16. DOI: 10.1017/S0007114510000218

[83] Ohgami K, Ilieva I, Shiratori K, Koyama Y, Jin X, Yoshida K, et al. Anti-inflammatory effects of aronia extract on rat endotoxin-induced uveitis. Investigative Ophthalmology & Visual Science. 2005;**46**:275-281. DOI: 10.1167/iovs.04-0715

[84] Varadinova M, Docheva-Drenska D, Boyadjieva N. Effects of anthocyanins on learning and memory of ovariectomized rats. Menopause. 2009;**16**:345-349. DOI: 10.1097/gme.0b013e3181847619

[85] Chang S, Cassidy A, Willett W, Rimm E, O'Reilly E, Okereke O. Dietary flavonoid intake and risk of incident depression in midlife and older women. The American Journal of Clinical Nutrition. 2016;**104**:704-714. DOI: 10.3945/ajcn.115.124545

[86] Khalid S, Barfoot K, May G, Lamport D, Reynolds S, Williams C. Effects of acute blueberry flavonoids on mood in children and young adults. Nutrients. 2017;**9**:158. DOI: 10.3390/nu9020158

[87] Nabavi S, Khan H, D'onofrio G, Šamec D, Shirooie S, Dehpour S, et al. Pigenin as neuroprotective agent: Of mice and men. Pharmacological Research. 2018;**128**:359-365. DOI: 10.1016/j.phrs.2018.10.008

[88] Di Lorenzo A, Sobolev A, Nabavi S, Sureda A, Moghaddam A, Khanjani S, et al. Post-stroke depression: Antidepressive effects of a chemically characterized maqui berry extract in a mouse model (*Aristotelia chilensis* (molina) stuntz). Food and Chemical Toxicology. 2019;**129**:434-443. DOI: 10.1016/j.fct.2019.04.023

[89] Gutierres J, Carvalho F, Schetinger M, Marisco P, Agostinho P, Rodrigues M, et al. Anthocyanins restore behavioral and biochemical changes caused by streptozotocin-induced sporadic dementia of Alzheimer's type. Life Sciences. 2014;**96**:7-17. DOI: 10.1016/j.lfs.2013.11.014

[90] McNamara R, Kalt W, Shidler M, McDonald J, Summer S, Stein A, et al. Cognitive response to fish oil, blueberry, and combined supplementation in older adults with subjective cognitive impairment. Neurobiology of Aging. 2018;**64**:147-156. DOI: 10.1016/j.neurobiolaging.2017.12.003

[91] Fan D, Alamri Y, Liu K, MacAskill M, Harris P, Brimble M, et al. Supplementation of blackcurrant anthocyanins increased cyclic glycine-proline in the cerebrospinal fluid of parkinson patients: Potential treatment to improve insulin-like growth factor-1 function. Nutrients. 2018;**10**:714. DOI: 10.3390/nu10060714

[92] Qian F, Wang M, Wang J, Lu C. Anthocyanin-rich blueberry extract ameliorates the behavioral deficits of MPTP-induced mouse model of Parkinson's disease via anti-oxidative mechanisms. YM. 2019;**3**:72-78. DOI: 10.4236/ym.2019.31008

[93] Devore E, Kang J, Breteler M, Grodstein F. Dietary intakes of berries and flavonoids in relation to cognitive decline. Annals of Neurology. 2012;**72**:135-143. DOI: 10.1002/ana.23594

[94] Watson A, Haskell-Ramsay C, Kennedy D, Cooney J, Trower T, Scheepens A. Acute supplementation with blackcurrant extracts modulates cognitive functioning and inhibits monoamine oxidase-B in healthy young adults. Journal of Functional Foods. 2015;**17**:524-539. DOI: 10.1016/j.jff.2015.06.005

[95] Whyte A, Williams C. Effects of a single dose of a flavonoid-rich blueberry drink on memory in 8 to 10 y old children. Nutrition. 2015;**31**:531-534. DOI: 10.1016/j.nut.2014.09.013

[96] Clauss J, Avery S, Benningfield M, Blackford J. Social anxiety is associated with BNST's response to unpredictability. Depression and Anxiety. 2019;**36**:666-675. DOI: 10.1002/da.22891

[97] WHO. Depression and Other Common Mental Disorders Global Health Estimates. 2017. Available from: http://apps.who.int/iris/bitstream/10665/254610/1/WHO-MSD-MER-2017.2-eng.pdf [Accessed: 02 August 2019]

[98] Lakhan S, Vieira K. Nutritional and herbal supplements for anxiety and anxiety-related disorders: Systematic review. Nutrition Journal. 2010;**9**:42. DOI: 10.1186/1475-2891-9-42

[99] Carlini E. Plants and the central nervous system. Pharmacology, Biochemistry, and Behavior. 2003;**75**:501-512. DOI: 10.1016/S0091-3057(03)00112-6

[100] Ravindran L, Stein M. The pharmacologic treatment of anxiety disorders: A review of progress. The Journal of Clinical Psychiatry. 2010;**71**:839-854. DOI: 10.4088 / JCP.10r06218blu

[101] Viola R, Brennan R, Davies H, Sommerville L. L-ascorbic acid accumulation in berries of *Ribes nigrum* L. The Journal of Horticultural Science and Biotechnology. 2000;**75**: 409-412. DOI: 10.1080/14620316.2000.11511260

[102] Valcheva-Kuzmanova S, Zhelyazkova-Savova M. Anxiolytic-like effect of *Aronia gmelanocarpa* fruit juice in rats. Methods and Findings in Experimental and Clinical Pharmacology. 2009;**31**:651-654. DOI: 10.1358/mf.2009.31.10.1423884

[103] Días A, Rozet E, Chataigné G, Oliveira A, Rabelo C, Hubert P, et al. A rapid validated UHPLC-PDA method for anthocyanins quantification from Euterpe oleracea fruits. Journal of Chromatography B. 2012;**907**:108-116. DOI: 10.1016/j.jchromb.2012.09.015

[104] Tomić M, Ignjatović Đ, Tovilović-Kovačević G, Krstić-Milošević D, Ranković S, Popović T, et al. Reduction of an xiety-like and depression-like behaviors in rats after one month of drinking Aronia melanocarpa berry juice. Food & Function. 2016;**7**:3111-3120. DOI: 10.1039/c6fo00321d

[105] Eftimov M, Valcheva-Kuzmanova S. Antidepressant-like effect of Aronia melanocarpa fruit juice applied subchronically to rats. Scripta Scientifica Medica. 2013;**45**:7-11. DOI: 10.14748/ssm.v45i1.990

[106] Valcheva-Kuzmanova S, Eftimov M, Belcheva I, Belcheva S, Tashev R. Anti-anxiety effect of *Aronia melanocarpa* fruit juice administered subchronically to rats. Farmácia. 2016;**64**:367-371. DOI: 10.1358/mf.2009.31.10.1423884

[107] Valcheva-Kuzmanova S, Blagović B, Valić S. Electron spin resonance measurement of radical scavenging activity of *Aronia melanocarpa* fruit juice. Pharmacognosy Magazine. 2012;**8**:171. DOI: 10.4103/0973-1296.96583

[108] RiazM,Zia-Ul-HaqM,Ur-RahmanN, Ahmad M. Neuropharmacological effects of methanolic extracts of *Rubus fruticosus* L. Turkish Journal of Medical Sciences. 2014;**44**:454-460. DOI: 10.3906/sag-1211-1

[109] Nogueira E, Rosa G, Haraguchi M, Vassilieff V. Anxiolytic effect of *Rubus brasilensis* in rats and mice. Journal of Ethnopharmacology. 1998;**61**:111-117. DOI: 10.1016/S0378-8741(98)00022-1

[110] Zanoli P, Avallone R, Baraldi M. Behavioral characterisation of the

flavonoids apigenin and chrysin. Fitoterapia. 2000;**71**:117-123. DOI: 10.1016/S0367-326X (00)00186-6

[111] Kessler R. The costs of depression. Psychiatric Clinics of North America. 2012;**35**:1-14. DOI: 10.1016/j.psc.2011.11.005

[112] Hammer J, Toland M. Internal structure and reliability of the internalized stigma of mental illness scale (ISMI-29) and brief versions (ISMI-10, ISMI-9) among Americans with depression. Stigma and Health. 2017;**2**:159. DOI: 10.1037/sah0000049

[113] Kok R, Reynolds C. Management of depression in older adults. Journal of the American Medical Association. 2017;**317**:2114. DOI: 10.1001/jama.2017.570

[114] Campbell S, MacQueen G. The role of the hippocampus in the pathophysiology of major depression. Journal of Psychiatry & Neuroscience. 2004;**29**:417-426. DOI: 10.1037/t01554-000

[115] Malberg J, Eisch A, Nestler E, Duman R. Chronic antidepressant treatment increases neurogenesis in adult rat hippocampus. The Journal of Neuroscience. 2000;**20**:9104-9110. DOI: 10.1523/JNEUROSCI.20-24-09104.2000

[116] Finberg J, Rabey J. Inhibitors of MAO-A and MAO-B in psychiatry and neurology. Frontiers in Pharmacology. 2016;**7**:340. DOI: 10.3389/fphar.2016.00340

[117] Heppner F, Ransohoff R, Becher B. Immune attack: The role of inflammation in Alzheimer disease. Nature Reviews. Neuroscience. 2015;**16**:358-372. DOI: 10.1038/nrn3880

[118] Mayeux R, Stern Y. Epidemiology of Alzheimer disease. Cold Spring Harbor Perspectives in Medicine. 2012;**2**:1-18. DOI: 10.1101/cshperspect.a006239

[119] Raskin J, Cummings J, Hardy J, Schuh K, Dean RA. Neurobiology of Alzheimer's disease: Integrated molecular, physiological, anatomical, biomarker, and cognitive dimensions. Current Alzheimer Research. 2015;**12**:712-722. DOI: 10.2174/1567205012666150701103107

[120] Kim G, Kim J, Rhie S, Yoon S. The role of oxidative stress in neurodegenerative diseases. Experimental Neurobiology. 2015;**24**:325-340. DOI: 10.5607/en.2015.24.4.325

[121] Cervellati C, Wood P, Romani A, Valacchi G, Squerzanti M, Sanz J, et al. Oxidative challenge in Alzheimer's disease: State of knowledge and future needs. Journal of Investigative Medicine. 2016;**64**:21-32. DOI: 10.1136/jim-2015-000017

[122] Huang W, Zhang X, Chen W. Role of oxidative stress in Alzheimer's disease (review). Biomedical Reports. 2016;**4**:519-522. DOI: 10.3892/br.2016.630

[123] Figueira I, Tavares L, Jardim C, Costa I, Terrasso A, Almeida A, et al. Blood-brain barrier transport and neuroprotective potential of blackberry-digested polyphenols: An in vitro study. European Journal of Nutrition. 2019;**58**:113-130. DOI: 10.1007/s00394-017-1576-y

[124] Vepsäläinen S, Koivisto H, Pekkarinen E. Anthocyanin-enriched bilberry and blackcurrant extractsmodulate amyloid precursor protein processing and alleviate behavioral abnormalities in the APP/PS1 mouse model of Alzheimer's disease. Journal of Nutritional Biochemistry. 2013;**24**:360-370. DOI: 10.1016/j.jnutbio.2012.07.006

[125] Dai J, Patel J, Mumper R. Characterization of blackberry extract and its antiproliferative and

antiinflammatory properties. Journal of Medicinal Food. 2007;**10**:258-650. DOI: 10.1089/jmf.2006.238

[126] Shukitt-Hale B, Cheng V, Mint JJ. Effects of blackberries on motor andcognitive function in aged rats. Nutritional Neuroscience. 2009;**12**:135-140. DOI: 10.1179/147683009X423292

[127] Pacheco S, Soares M, Gutierres J, Gerzson M, Carvalho F, Azambuja J, et al. Anthocyanins as a potential pharmacological agent to manage memory deficit, oxidative stress and alterations in ion pump activity induced by experimental sporadic dementia of Alzheimer's type. The Journal of Nutritional Biochemistry. 2018;**56**:193-204. DOI: 10.1016/j.jnutbio.2018.02.014

[128] Van Mae le-Fabry G, Hoet P, Vilain F, Lison D. Occupational exposure to pesticides and Parkinson's disease: A systematic review and meta-analysis of cohort studies. Environment International. 2012;**46**:30-43. DOI: 10.1016/j.envint.2012.05.004

[129] de Lau L, Breteler M. Epidemiology of Parkinson's disease. Journal of Neural Transmission. 2006;**124**:525-535. DOI: 10.1007/s00702-017-1686-y

[130] Costa J, Lunet N, Santos C, Santos J, Vaz-Carneiro A. Caffeine exposure and the risk of Parkinson's disease: A systematic review and meta-analysis of observational studies. Journal of Alzheimer's Disease. 2010;**20**:221-238. DOI: 10.3233/JAD-2010-091525

[131] Connolly B, Lang A. Pharmacological treatment of parkinson disease: A review. Journal of the American Medical Association. 2014;**311**:1670-1683. DOI: 10.1001/jama.2014.3654

[132] Bronstein J, Tagliati M, Alterman R, Lozano A, Volkmann J, Stefani A. Deep brain stimulation for Parkinson disease: An expert consensus and review of key issues. Archives of Neurology. 2011;**68**:165. DOI: 10.1001/archneurol.2010.260

[133] Grosso C, Valentão P, Ferreres F, Andrade P. The use of flavonoids in central nervous system disorders. Current Medicinal Chemistry. 2013;**20**:694-719. DOI: 10.2174/0929867311320990155

[134] Chen L, Xin X, Yuan Q, Su D, Liu W. Phytochemical properties and antioxidant capacities of various colored berries. Journal of Science and Food Agriculture. 2014;**94**:180-188. DOI: 10.1002/jsfa.6216

[135] Strathearn K, Yousef G, Grace M, Roy S, Tambe M, Ferruzzi M, et al. Neuroprotective effects of anthocyanin- and proanthocyanidin-rich extracts in cellular models of Parkinson's disease. Brain Research. 2014;**1555**:60-77. DOI: 10.1016/j.brainres.2014.01.047

[136] Kao A, Racine C, Quitania L, Kramer J, Christine C, Miller L. Cognitive and neuropsychiatric profile of the synucleinopathies: Parkinson's disease, dementia with Lewy bodies and multiple system atrophy. Alzheimer Disease and Associated Disorders. 2009;**23**:365-370. DOI: 10.1097/WAD.0b013e3181b5065d

[137] Milbury P, Kalt W. Xenobiotic metabolism and berry flavonoid transport across the blood-brain barrier. Journal of Agricultural and Food Chemistry. 2010;**58**:3950-3956. DOI: 10.1021/jf903529m

[138] Del Rio D, Rodriguez-Mateos A, Spencer J, Tognolini M, Borges G, Crozier A. Dietary (poly) phenolics in human health: Structures, bioavailability, and evidence of protective effects against chronic diseases. Antioxidants & Redox

Signaling. 2013;**18**:1818-1892. DOI: 10.1089/ars.2012.4581

[139] Forno L, Langston J, DeLanney L, Irwin I, Ricaurte G. Locus ceruleus lesions and eosinophilic inclusions in MPTP-treated monkeys. Annals of Neurology. 1986;**20**:449-455. DOI: 10.1002/ana.410200403

[140] Kopin I, Markey S. MPTP toxicity: Implications for research in Parkinson's disease. Annual Review of Neuroscience. 1988;**11**:81-96. DOI: 10.1002/ana.410200403

[141] Heikkila R, Sieber B, Manzino L, Sonsalla P. Some features of the nigrostriatal dopaminergic neurotoxin 1-methyl-4-phenyl-1, 2, 3, 6-tetrahydropyridine (MPTP) in the mouse. Molecular and Chemical Neuropathology. 1989;**10**:171-183. DOI: 10.1007/BF03159727

[142] Calon F, Lavertu N, Lemieux A, Morissette M, Goulet M, Grondin R, et al. Effect of MPTP-induced denervation on basal ganglia GABAB receptors: Correlation with dopamine concentrations and dopamine transporter. Synapse. 2001;**40**:225-234. DOI: 10.1002/syn.1045

[143] Blanchet J, Longpré F, Bureau G, Morissette M, DiPaolo T, Bronchti G, et al. Resveratrol, a red wine polyphenol, protects dopaminergic neurons in MPTP-treated mice. Progress in Neuro-Psychopharmacology and Biological Psychiatry. 2008;**32**:1243-1250. DOI: 10.1016/j.pnpbp.2008.03.024

[144] Haskell-Ramsay C, Stuart R, Okello E, Watson A. Cognitive and mood improvements following acute supplementation with purple grape juice in healthy young adults. European Journal of Nutrition. 2017;**56**:2621-2631. DOI: 10.1007/s00394-017-1541-9

[145] Krikorian R, Boespflug E, Fleck D, Stein A, Wightman J, Shidler M, et al. Concord grape juice supplementation and neurocognitive function in human aging. Journal of Agricultural and Food Chemistry. 2012;**60**:5736-5742. DOI: doi.org/10.1021/jf300277g

[146] Lamport D, Lawton C, Merat N, Jamson H, Myrissa K, Hofman D, et al. Concord grape juice, cognitive function, and driving performance: A 12-wk, placebo-controlled, randomized crossover trial in mothers of preteen children. The American Journal of Clinical Nutrition. 2016;**103**:775-783. DOI: 10.3945/ajcn.115.114553

[147] Whyte A, Schafer G, Williams C. Cognitive effects following acute wild blueberry supplementation in 7- to 10-year-old children. European Journal of Nutrition. 2016;**55**:2151-2162. DOI: 10.1007/s00394-015-1029

[148] Miller M, Hamilton D, Joseph J, Shukitt-Hale B. Dietary blueberry improves cognition among older adults in a randomized, double-blind, placebo-controlled trial. European Journal of Nutrition. 2018;**57**:1169-1180. DOI: 10.1007/s00394-017-1400-8

[149] Dove A, Pollmann S, Schubert T, Wiggins C, von Cramon D. Prefrontal cortex activation in task switching: An eventrelated fMRI study. Cognitive Brain Research. 2000;**9**:103-109. DOI: 10.1016/s0926-6410(99)00029-4

[150] Kent K, Charlton K, Roodenrys S, Batterham M, Potter J, Traynor V, et al. Consumption of anthocyanin-rich cherry juice for 12 weeks improves memory and cognition in older adults with mild-to-moderate dementia. European Journal of Nutrition. 2017;**56**:333-341. DOI: 10.1007/s00394-015-1083-y

[151] Whyte A, Cheng N, Fromentin E, Williams C. A randomized, double-blinded, placebo-controlled study to compare the safety and efficacy of

low dose enhanced wild blueberry powder and wild blueberry extract (ThinkBlue™) in maintenance of episodic and working memory in older adults. Nutrients. 2018;**10**:1-14. DOI: 10.3390/nu10060660

[152] Barfoot K, May G, Lamport D, Ricketts J, Riddell P, Williams C. The effects of acute wild blueberry supplementation on the cognition of 7-10-year-old schoolchildren. European Journal of Nutrition. 2019;**58**:2911-2920. DOI: 10.1007/s00394-018-1843-6

[153] Bell L, Williams C. A pilot dose-response study of the acute effects of haskap berry extract (*Lonicera caerulea* L.) on cognition, mood, and blood pressure in older adults. European Journal of Nutrition. 2018;**58**:3325-3334. DOI: 10.1007/s00394-018-1877-9

[154] Rodriguez-Mateos A, Rendeiro C, Bergillos-Meca T, Tabatabaee S, George T, Heiss C, et al. Intake and time dependence of blueberry flavonoid-induced improvements in vascular function: A randomized, controlled, double-blind, crossover intervention study with mechanistic insights into biological activity. The American Journal of Clinical Nutrition. 2013:1179-1191. DOI: 10.3945/ajcn.113.066639

[155] Gandhi S, Abramov A. Mechanism of oxidative stress in neurodegeneration. Oxidative Medicine and Cellular Longevity. 2012;**2012**:1-11. DOI: 10.1155/2012/428010

[156] Walton J, Selvakumar B, Weil Z, Snyder S, Nelson R. Neuronal nitric oxide synthase and NADPH oxidase interact to affect cognitive, affective, and social behaviors in mice. Behavioural Brain Research. 2013;**256**:320-327. DOI: 10.1016/j.bbr.2013.08.003

[157] Williams C, Dodd G, Lamport D, Spencer J, Butler L. Effects of anthocyanin-rich blueberries on cognitive function in healthy younger and older adults. Innovation in Aging. 2017;**1**:1362. DOI: 10.1093/geroni/igx004.5009

[158] Hornfeldt C, Collins J. Toxicity of nightshade berries (*Solanum dulcamara*) in mice 1, 2. Journal of Toxicology: Clinical Toxicology. 1990;**28**:185-192. DOI: 10.3109/15563659008993491

[159] Kees M, Beckel N, Sharp C. Successful treatment of *Solanum dulcamara* intoxication in a Labrador retriever puppy. The Canadian Veterinary Journal. 2015;**56**:1283-1286. DOI: 10.3109/15563659008993491

[160] Woldemeskel M, Styer E. Feeding behavior-related toxicity due to Nandina domestica in cedar waxwings (*Bombycilla cedrorum*). Veterinary Medicine International. 2010;**2010**:1-4. DOI: 10.4061/2010/818159

[161] Huang W, Zhang H, Liu W, Li C. Survey of antioxidant capacity and phenolic composition of blueberry, blackberry, and strawberry in Nanjing. Journal of Zhejiang University. Science. B. 2012;**13**:94-102. DOI: 10.1631/jzus.B1100137

[162] Luís Â, Duarte A, Pereira L, Domingues F. Interactions between the major bioactive polyphenols of berries: Effects on antioxidant properties. European Food Research and Technology. 2018;**244**:175-185. DOI: 10.1007/s00217-017-2948-5

Chapter 4

Pharmaceutical and Botanical Management of Pain Associated with Psychopathology: A Narrative Review

Minerva Hernández Lozano,
Marcos Fernando Ocaña Sánchez,
Rosa Virginia García Rodríguez, Van Dan Castro Gerónimo,
Libna Sulem Gallardo Beatriz,
Ibrahim Guillermo Castro Torres,
María Gabriela Alcántara López, Julio César González Ortiz,
Gabriela Josefina Mendoza Rangel
and Tania Monserrat Camacho Márquez

Abstract

Generally, pain can be described as an unpleasant sensory or emotional experience associated with tissue damage. Chronic pain has become a public health problem because among 35 and 75% of the world population has shown the symptom. In particular, neuropathic pain has shown high comorbidity disorders such as anxiety and depression. Conventional therapies for treating pain include nonsteroidal anti-inflammatory drugs (NSAIDs), corticosteroids, tricyclic antidepressants, anticonvulsants, and opioids, which usually cause some side effects such as gastritis, headache, liver and kidney toxicity, and drug dependence. Conventional pharmaceuticals also tend to be expensive, and they cannot be easily afforded in developing countries, which have led to the use of natural products as an alternative treatment. In this chapter, we reviewed the current research of natural products for pain treatment. We also describe preclinical studies that assess the effect of some natural products on pain therapy, phytochemistry research, toxicity, adverse effects, and biosecurity. We also describe how conventional pain is managed and the possible use of compounds obtained from vegetable species for pain treatment.

Keywords: pain, analgesic, anti-inflammatory, herbal medicine, phytopharmaceuticals

1. Introduction

Over the course of history, the pain has been manifested in a wide range of forms, and it has not been treated properly. It is estimated that approximately 116 million

Kind of drug	Type of pain	Examples	Doses	Side effect
NSAIDs	Nociceptive	Acetaminophen	325–1000 mg PO every 4–6 h; max dose 4 g per day	GI irritation, renal, and hepatic dysfunction
		Diclofenac	50 mg PO every 8 h; max dose 150 mg per day	GI irritation, bleeding, hepatic, and renal dysfunction
		Ibuprofen	200–400 mg PO every 6 h; 1.2 g per day	GI irritation, bronchospasm, bleeding, and renal dysfunction
		Naproxen	250 mg PO every 6–8 h; max dose 1 g per day	GI irritation, bleeding, renal dysfunction, and bronchospasm
		Indomethacin	25 mg PO every 8–12 h; max dose 100 mg per day	GI irritation, renal, and hepatic dysfunction
Opiates	Nociplastic/ neuropathic	Tramadol	25–50 mg PO every 6–8 h; max dose 400 mg per day	Dizziness, drowsiness, nausea, dry mouth, vomiting, and constipation
		Morphine	10–15 mg PO 3–6 h; 0.1 mg/kg IV	Nausea, vomiting, drowsiness, constipation, and sedation
		Oxycodone	5–10 mg PO every 3–6 h	Constipation, nausea, vomiting, drowsiness, dry mouth, hallucinations, and delirium
		Hydromorphone	2–4 mg PO; 0.25–0.5 mg/kg every 6 h	Pruritus, nausea, and rapid sedation
		Fentanyl	0.5 mcg/kg	Blurred vision, nausea, confusion, dizziness, and irregular heartbeats
Anticonvulsants	Nociplastic/ neuropathic	Gabapentin	Stepwise increase every 3–5 days from 300 mg to 1200 PO every 8 h; max dose 3.6 g per day	Fatigue, ataxia, nystagmus, weight gain, and dizziness
		Pregabalin	50–75 mg PO every 12 h	Dizziness, fatigue, weight gain, and thrombocytopenia
		Phenytoin	100 mg PO every 12 h; max dose 200 mg per day	Nausea, vomiting, constipation, dizziness, drowsiness, trouble sleeping, or nervousness
Antidepressants	Neuropathic	Amitriptyline	Stepwise increase every 7–10 days from 25 mg to 50 PO every 6 h; max dose 200 mg per day	Vomiting, nausea, diarrhea, mouth pain, unusual taste, weight gain, urinary retention, and rash
		Venlafaxine	Stepwise increase every day from 75–150 mg PO every 8 h; max dose 150 mg per day	Libido reduction, loss of appetite, nausea or vomiting, constipation, dry mouth, trouble sleeping, and lack of energy
		Mirtazapine	Stepwise increase every 2 weeks from 15 to 45 mg PO a day; max dose 45 mg per day	Dry mouth, drowsiness, constipation weight gain, weakness, lack of energy, and dizziness

DOI: http://dx.doi.org/10.5772/intechopen.91154

Kind of drug	Type of pain	Examples	Doses	Side effect
Others	Neuropathic	Ketamine	0.115–0.3 mg/kg IV	Nausea or vomiting, agitation, dizziness, and a sensation of unreality
		Propofol	30–40 mg IV repeating 10 mg every 3–5 min; max dose 120 mg per day	Hypotension, sedation, respiratory depression, and hypertriglyceridemia
		Capsaicin	Cream: 3–4 times per day; patches: one time a day and repeated as often as every 3 months	Burning, dryness, itching, redness, swelling, or soreness at the application site

PO, per os rout; IV, intravenous rout; GI, gastrointestinal.

Table 1.
Drugs used in acute and chronic pain.

Americans have experienced chronic pain, which is higher than those affected by chronic diseases, such as heart disease, cancer, and diabetes, among others. The simplest way to classify pain is based on its intensity as mild, moderate, and severe or using a scale from 0 to 10, where 0 is the lowest and 10 the highest. Other scales that are typically used are the unimodal scale such as the Analog Verbal Scale (AVS), the Visual Analog Scale (VAS), and the Numerical Scale (NS), among others. These scales are somewhat informal because pain is not easy to measure. Therefore, variations might affect critical evaluation when pain is manifested in all forms. Some authors refer to the use of the one-dimensional test to reach a standardized measure of pain; however, the researcher must adjust the test depending on the type of pain and type of research.

Aspirin and morphine, which are derived from plants, have been widely used for analgesic purposes. These compounds belong to nonsteroidal anti-inflammatory (NSAIDs) and opiate drug groups, respectively, and they are the most used nowadays [1]. Once the pain evolves and becomes chronic, several types of oral neuromodulators are often included in the patient treatment, for example, certain anticonvulsants and antidepressants [2], see **Table 1**.

In 2012, the use of NSAIDs in North America represented 98 million of the total prescriptions, and more than 29 million adults were regular users of these medications. Furthermore, a study in Sweden showed that these types of medications were the most commonly prescribed oral analgesics for the musculoskeletal system, with 79% of prescriptions for a period of 5 years [3]. Opioid consumption causes side effects such as physical dependence, tolerance, and addiction, while NSAIDs cause intestinal disorders and ulceration [4]. Because the long-term pain treatment with conventional medicine is expensive and people commonly know the side effects that these may cause, patients tend to look at alternative drugs, most of the times based on herbal treatments. However, patients do not inform the use of natural products to their physicians, which may lead to potential health problems caused by pharmacological interactions with other drugs prescribed. This represents a relevant issue in countries where the use of plants is common but not necessarily regulated [5]. In the search for new effective and safe alternatives to treat several processes of pain, natural resources have been a relevant option for current medicine. Considering that pain is one of the most persistent and disabling manifestations present in several diseases, it has been increasingly becoming a major health problem, and it is also a challenge for modern medicine. Therefore, it is necessary to fully understand the pathophysiology of pain as well as alternatives that might be effective for treating it.

2. Pain classification, semiology, and diagnosis

The International Association for the Study of Pain (IASP) defines pain as "an unpleasant sensory and emotional experience associated with actual or potential tissue damage or described in terms of such damage" [6]. Each person reacts differently to a pain stimulus, even before similar situations and injuries. Since pain is learned and sensed from the early stages of life, how people describe is often related to a particular personal experience including a patient's culture, traumatic experiences, mood, biological aspects, and genetics. The words "pain" and "suffering" have often been used as synonyms, but the experience of suffering has been differentiated from pain. Suffering has been defined not only as a complement to the pain experience but also as vulnerability, dehumanization, a lost sense of self, lack of control over time and space, and the inability to find a meaning or purpose of the painful experience. The term "suffering" conveys the experience of pain beyond sensory attributes [7].

There are several ways to classify pain. The most common classification considers aspects such as origin, duration, neurophysiological characteristics, and intensity.

Based on its origin, pain could be oncological and nononcological. Oncological pain is caused by a cancerous process (invasion, understanding, infiltration, obstruction, etc.), associated with therapy (chemotherapy, radiotherapy, etc.), acute pain caused by diagnostic procedures (lumbar puncture, pleurodesis, embolization, opioid-induced hyperalgesia, etc.), and that is associated with neoplastic or related pathology (vertebral collapse, intratumoral hemorrhage, myalgia associated with sepsis, etc.) [8]. Noncancer pain is classified based on its duration as acute and chronic. The first one is limited to the time duration of fewer than 3 months. Noncancer pain has a little psychological component and usually affects somatic or visceral structures. By contrast, chronic pain has an unlimited duration, lasting more than 3 months. Chronic pain differs from acute pain in the pathophysiological mechanisms and in its temporality in which the adaptive physiological process that characterizes is shown [9–11]. In 2019, a new classification of chronic pain was proposed by the World Health Organization (ICD-11) [12], according to its neurophysiological characteristics, as nociceptive, neuropathic, and nociplastic [6, 12], see **Table 2**.

Recently, an international multidisciplinary research group proposed to the scientific community a fifth definition of pain called mixed pain, which is produced by a complex overlap of the different types of pain known (nociceptive, neuropathic, and nociplastic) in any combination, acting simultaneously and/or concurrently to cause pain in the same area of the body, either acutely or chronic [13]. This difficulty of evaluating pain makes possible to resort to instruments that, with the minimum effort of the patient, are easily understandable, reliable, and valid.

Type of pain	Nociceptive		Neuropathic	Nociplastic
Origin	**Somatic**	**Visceral**	**Central nervous system**	**Neurophysiologic**
Receptors	Cutaneous or deep tissues such as skin, muscles, tendons, fascia, bones, or periosteum nociceptors	Walls of abdominal viscera nociceptors	Produced by dysfunction or injury to peripheral nerve pathways in the absence of demonstrable tissue damage	Peripheral receptors or injury of the somatosensory system
Characteristics	Specific localization stabbing, acute, or chronic and shows periods of exacerbation with variable intensity depending on the inducing stimulus	Deep, spastic, and oppressive, poorly located or may be referred to as cutaneous surface distant from the origin of pain	Stabbing, burning, paroxysmal accompanied by paresthesia, dysesthesia, hyperalgesia, and allodynia, with a sensory deficit	Altered nociception even though there is no clear evidence of actual or potential tissue damage
Examples	Burns, bumps, bruises, sprains, and bone fractures	Shoulder pain in myocardial infarction	Postherpetic neuralgia, carpal tunnel syndrome, peripheral neuropathy, and phantom limb pain	Fibromyalgia, chronic fatigue, vulvodynia, and interstitial cystitis

Table 2.
Classification of the chronic pain according to the World Health Organization.

These include the McGill Pain Questionnaire (MPQ), Lattinen Test, Spanish Pain Questionnaire (CDE), Chronic Pain Coping Questionnaire (CAD), West Haven-Yale Multidimensional Pain Inventory (WHYMPI), Brief Pain Inventory, and the scales of assessment of neuropathic pain: the LANSS Pain Scale, the Neuropathic Pain Questionnaire (NPQ), Questionnaire DN4 (DN4), and Pain DETECT, among others [14]. It is important to note that the purpose of these tests is to assist the clinicians in assessing the severity of the pain or its causes. Tests correctly classify the patients as suffering from nociceptive and neuropathic pain.

3. Pain epidemiology

Epidemiological studies have shown that in the last month approximately half of people will have experienced an episode of pain that lasted at least 1 day, and the most common sites reported, in a study in the UK population, were the part lower back (30%), hip (25%), neck and shoulder (25%), and knee (24%) [15]. According to the US Institute of Medicine, 80% of patients who undergo surgery report postoperative pain, and 88% of these patients indicate moderate, severe, or extreme pain levels, if improperly managed between 10 and 60% of them will develop persistent pain postoperative [16].

Concerning to oncologic pain, a systemic review that covered the period from 1966 to 2005 documented that the prevalence of pain after curative procedures of cancer pathology was 33% (95% CI 21–46%). While in those who were managed with anticancer therapy, pain occurred in 59% (CI 44–73%); in those with an advanced, terminal disease and with metastasis in 64% (CI 58–69%) and patients with any disease status in 53% (CI 43–63%). Of the patients with pain, more than a third presented moderate to severe intensity, with a high prevalence in patients with head and neck cancer (70%; 95% CI 51–88%) [8]. To chronic pain, the higher prevalence was unemployed, people without one university degree who live in poverty or rural areas. About the prevalence by sex and age, women and the elderly showed an elevation of this kind of pain [17].

Regarding the bad management of acute pain, there is a risk that a chronic painful syndrome will develop, with all its consequences for the patient, for his family and his environment. The chronicity of pain commonly involves anxiety, depression, fatigue, cognitive difficulty, and insomnia. Functional limitations and the consequent absence from work have been considered as part of the impact on the quality of life of high-impact diseases. It is currently known that people with chronic pain are more likely to have disabilities than those without pain. In addition, this disability is more likely in this condition than in any chronic health condition, including stroke, kidney failure, cancer, diabetes, and heart disease. The impact in terms of work absenteeism is evident both for the individual (loss of self-esteem, income, and low quality of life) and for the society (loss of productivity and higher health care expense) [18].

Pain is a major global public health problem because it has an important social and economic impact. It is necessary to have a clear understanding of the types of sensory signs and symptoms that should be assessed as pain since it is an individual and subjective experience.

4. Pain comorbidity

The pain usually accompanies various diseases, such as organ failure or mental disorder. A high number of patients with a mental disorder show some type of pain, but not all have any significant physical injury to justify such pain [19]. The relationship between chronic pain and psychiatric disorders in addition to comorbidity is that these disorders may arise the risk of chronic pain, as well as the pain can contribute to developing psychiatric disorders. Among the most common diseases with which it is related are anxiety, depression, dementia, and schizophrenia [20].

Pathological anxiety is one of the most common mental disorders. It is an emotion that is characterized by an exaggerated concern for future events or situations of uncertainty [21]. Anxiety disorder can affect the response of pain in various forms or states. A clinical study assayed on healthy female volunteers explored the effects of a particular type of anxiety (pain anxiety). The volunteer received electrocutaneous pain stimuli and the pain anxiety where measured by the Fear of Pain Questionnaire and Pain Anxiety Symptoms Scale. Three or six months later, the evaluated group was asked to rate the pain anxiety that they felt when the test was developed. It was demonstrated that pain anxiety can influence the memory of unpleasant experiences like experimental pain [22].

Anxiety is also common in diseases involving chronic pain stages such as multiple sclerosis and arthritis, in which anxiety disorder is more prevalent than in the general population. This psychiatric disorder also can contribute to the development and severity of symptoms of inflammatory arthritis [23]. A study conducted in patients (58% female, mean age 43) who were receiving opioid agonist therapy for chronic pain showed that the weekly practice of hatha yoga for 3 months can reduce the level of pain and perhaps mediated by the decrease of emotional symptoms such as anxiety [24].

Neuroanatomical correlates to the response to anxiety are very complex, involving various structures such as the medial prefrontal cortex, hypothalamic and amygdaloidal nuclei, the hippocampal formation, and the gray matter of the central portion of the midbrain. Patients with some anxiety disorder show a common pattern of activity of the hypothalamic-pituitary-adrenal (HPA) axis [21]. These areas are also related to the activation of the pain signaling pathway. On the other hand, when there is chronic pain, there is also hyperadrenalism and a decrease in the catecholaminergic pathway, as well as the activation of the HPA axis with continuous release of corticosteroid hormones. These alterations are also present in the population with some anxiety disorder and are prior to the onset of pain, so when activated, it works as a modulator for the response and activation of pain [25].

Depression is another mental illness that has grown in incidence and prevalence in recent years. This disorder is responsible for more lost each year than any other disorder, and this is mainly because many people suffer from this (about 350 million people worldwide) [26]. Patients with this disorder experience different types of pain, such as chronic pain, fibromyalgia, rheumatoid arthritis, headache, neck, abdominal, pelvic, and neuropathic pain [20], among others. Depression and pain share neurobiological pathways and neurotransmitters: depression is the result of an imbalance or functional deficiency of monoamines such as dopamine, serotonin, and norepinephrine. When these neurotransmitters decrease, the modulating effect of the GPA (periaqueductal gray) system is lost, which is the anatomical key to modulating pain or nociceptive pathway. When this happens, the lower body signals are amplified, and more emotions and attention are focused on it, that is why depressed patients report feeling pain in various body parts [27].

Dementia is a syndrome of damage or cognitive impairment that affects the lifestyle of people. The incidence of this disorder is high; it is estimated that in the world a new case of dementia occurs every 4 s. The most common form is associated with Alzheimer's disease in the elderly [28]. There are proposals on the mechanism that takes place to develop dementia, such as alterations in the immune system, cholesterol metabolism, endocytosis of neurotransmitters in the central nervous system, alterations in the vascular system, and frontotemporal lobar degeneration

(FTLD) [29]. Almost half of older people with dementia suffer any type of pain. Some of the most important changes related to dementia may arise cognitive domain of pain, such as alterations in semantic and episodic memory, executive function, and anticipation of it. Some studies have shown that dementia reduces the experience of pain, although what is suggested is that patients cannot recognize or remember this symptom [30]. Recognition of pain in people with this condition should be considered because it changes the quality of life of patients. If they cannot recognize the pain, or cannot to verbalize it, they will not be evaluated or treated properly [31].

Schizophrenia is another heterogeneous psychiatric disorder with a broad spectrum of clinical and biological manifestations. Patients with this disorder show structural changes in the brain, as well as the decreased volume of the hippocampus and cortex, and the lengthening of ventricular spaces. There are also changes in the organization and size of neurons and other brain cells. It has been shown that there are alterations in the dopaminergic and glutamatergic neurotransmission in the limbic system. On the other hand, peripheral molecular markers have been associated with developing this disease, such as IL-1β, IL-6, and TNF-α, which are known as pro-inflammatory cytokines [32]. With the release of these cytokines, an activation state of low-grade inflammation is reached, which worsens the prognosis of patients in relation to positive and negative psychotic symptoms, cognitive impairment, and loss of brain volume. In addition, an over activation of the HPA axis is observed, with a sustained release of cortisol [33]. One of the classic symptoms of schizophrenia, but which is not given much attention, is a pain without experimental provocation, including the percentage of people with this disease indicating which pain is not high. This may be due to reduced pain sensitivity in these patients produced by neuroanatomical alterations in the medial prefrontal and temporal areas of the brain since it is known that motivational-affective pain processing requires this intact neural circuit [34].

In summary, pain can modify the course of psychopathologies, as well as these conditions may alter the perception or memory pain (how it is recalled). Knowing how the neurobiological substrates in both (psychiatric disorders and pain) converge, help a better way to treat pathologies, and provide an opening to new forms and strategies to face or prevent them.

5. Conventional pain management

The pharmacological treatment of pain includes a wide range of medications, which mainly include nonsteroidal anti-inflammatory drugs (NSAIDs), opioids, antidepressants, and anticonvulsants. Classic NSAIDs were developed in the early 1900s, being the prototype the acetylsalicylic acid (aspirin), which possess antipyretic, anti-inflammatory, and analgesic actions. Subsequently, other molecules with similar activity were incorporated as paracetamol (acetaminophen), phenylbutazone, indomethacin, fenamates, naproxen, and ibuprofen [35, 36]. These drugs are prescribed for the management of inflammatory pain, and their analgesic effects of the latter are partly explained by reducing the biosynthesis of prostaglandins mediated by the inhibition of cyclooxygenase (COX), which leads to a reduction or reversal of peripheral sensitization. However, NSAIDs also modulate pain intensity by suppressing prostanoid biosynthesis in the central nervous system, thus affecting central sensitization [37].

The production of prostaglandins depends on the release of arachidonic acid, which in turn is released as a result of the action of phospholipase A2 on cell membrane phospholipids. The cyclooxygenase and lipoxygenase pathways represent the main routes for the oxidative metabolism of arachidonic acid. The catabolism of eicosanoic acid by cyclooxygenase produces cyclic prostaglandins. The peroxidation catalyzed by lipoxygenase gives rise to straight-chain hydroperoxyeicosatetraenoic acids (HPETEs), which may then be converted into hydroxyeicosatetraenoic acids (HETEs) and leukotrienes (LTs). Prostanoids (prostaglandins and thromboxane) do not activate nociceptors directly but sensitize them to both mechanical stimuli and other chemical mediators of nociception, such as bradykinin and histamine. However, stable E-series prostaglandins are clearly involved in the hyperalgesia observed in acute inflammation. Prostaglandin E2 (PGE2) is the predominant eicosanoid in many inflammatory conditions, acting synergistically with other mediators to sensitize receptors in afferent nerve endings to produce inflammatory pain. All NSAIDs inhibit the synthesis of prostaglandins at one or more points in the endoperoxide biosynthesis pathway. This unique property is a general characteristic and is believed to be the basis of their analgesic action [38].

Combinations of analgesics (Ketoprofen and Nefopam) with different mechanisms of action have been evaluated in distinct animal models of pain (acetic acid-induced writhing, formalin-induced licking in mice, induction of carrageenan unilateral hind-paw inflammation, and, induction of unilateral hind-paw incision in rat). Ketoprofen is an NSAID, which exhibits efficient antinociception in humans and animal models, particularly in inflammatory pain; its main mechanisms of action involve the inhibition of COX and lipoxygenase decreasing the production of prostaglandins and leukotrienes, respectively. On the other hand, Nefopam is an antinociceptive compound with both supraspinal and spinal sites of action, and its mechanism of action involves the inhibition of monoamine reuptake in the central nervous system; it increases the inhibiting tone of serotonergic and norepinephrine descending pathways by inhibiting the synaptosomal uptake of dopamine, norepinephrine, and serotonin. This study concluded that the co-administration is synergistic and should allow either to increase their analgesic efficacy or to reduce their side effects [39].

In a recent study of preclinical research, it was observed that pretreatment of male CF-1 mice with either clomipramine [1.0 mg/kg i.p. or 0.8 mg/kg intrathecal (i.t.)] or risperidone (0.01 mg/kg either i.p., as intrathecal) increased the antinociceptive potency of several NSAIDs, expressed by a decrease in the values of antinociceptive ED_{50} in a chemical model of inflammatory acute visceral pain, the abdominal acetic acid induced a writhing test in mouse. For the study, dose-response curves, i.p. or i.t., were performed to determine the ED_{50} of each of the NSAIDs: Ketoprofen (3, 10, 30, and 100 mg/kg, i.p. or 0.1, 0.3, 1, and 3 mg/kg, i.t.), Piroxicam (1, 3, 10, 30, and 100 mg/kg, i.p. or 0.1, 0.3, 1, and 3 mg/kg, i.t.), Nimesulide (1, 3, 10, and 30 mg/kg, i.p. or 0.03, 0.1, 0.3, and 1 mg/kg, i.t.), Parecoxib (0.3, 1, 3, and 10 mg/kg. i.p. or 0.1, 0.3, 1, and 3 mg/kg. i.t.), or Paracetamol (10, 30, 100, and 200 mg/kg, i.p. or 1, 3, 10, and 30 mg/kg, i.t.) [40].

Opioids are the main group of pharmacological therapies for pain. Useful guidelines for their administration have been developed for several clinical situations, including treatment of acute pain, trauma, cancer, nonmalignant chronic pain, and pain in children. In the case of cancer pain, adherence to standardized protocols can improve pain management significantly [41, 42]. Opioids should be prescribed concomitantly with other analgesics such as NSAIDs or paracetamol since they show a synergistic effect, and by reducing the dose of both, the possible adverse effects are reduced. This "opioid-sparing" strategy is the backbone of the "analgesic ladder" for pain management proposed by the WHO. If the intensity of pain is increased, weak-to-strong opioid medication can be adjusted, in which case they should be prescribed for continued dose or infusion, so that plasma levels remain stable and unnecessary suffering is avoided [4].

Gabapentinoids are recommended as first-line agents for neuropathic pain [43, 44]. Two examples of these substances are Pregabalin and Gabapentin not only used as an anticonvulsant but also prescribed to the management of postherpetic neuralgia without effects in painful sciatica [45]. Carbamazepine, Lamotrigine, and Oxcarbazepine are the first choice for the medical treatment of trigeminal neuralgia [46, 47]. They act as a dependent sodium channel blocker. Because of the unexpected drug interactions caused by a reduction in the activity of various hepatic cytochrome P450 enzymes that affect drug metabolism, carbamazepine is not recommended to treat any other types of neuropathic pain [44].

The first-line drugs to neuropathic pain include tricyclic antidepressants (TCAs) and selective serotonin-norepinephrine reuptake inhibitors (SSNRI). TCAs are recommended based on efficacy, safety, toxic effects, and cost [44]; they are efficacious for several types of neuropathic pain including diabetic peripheral neuropathy (DPN), nerve injury pain, PHN, and central post-stroke pain. The analgesic effects of TCAs are related to inhibiting the reuptake of noradrenaline and serotonin from presynaptic terminals [48]. Amitriptyline is the TCAs most prescribed in many circumstances where neuropathic pain is presented as central pain, DPN, and PHN [44]. SSNRIs, such as Venlafaxine and Duloxetine, are an effective drug in the treatment of neuropathic pain [49, 50]. They are mainly studied on painful polyneuropathy.

In recent years, connexins (Cxs) have been studied as targets for the development of new analgesic drugs. Connexins are a family of proteins with 20 subtypes and function as channels, junctions between cells, and hemichannels that sample the extracellular space and release substances such as neurotransmitters. One of the Cxs, Cx43, is expressed in astrocytes at the level of the central and peripheral nervous system. This has been studied in animal models and related to the genesis and maintenance of chronic pain, so it could be a promising therapeutic target for future treatments that act as Cx43-gap junction blockers, at the level of the trigeminal ganglion and the sciatic nerve [51].

6. Side effects and toxicity in pain pharmacotherapy

NSAIDs can promote various degrees of toxicity related to their pharmacokinetic and pharmacodynamic properties [11]. Its long-term use is a leading cause of morbidity especially in patients with risk factors, such as peptic ulcer and myocardial infarction, among others. The administration of these drugs or paracetamol frequently produces adverse effects such as gastrointestinal bleeding, hypertension, risk of infarction, hepatotoxicity, and renal failure [52–55]. Up to 25% of patients treated with NSAIDs have sodium retention, resulting in weight gain and developing peripheral edema. Likewise, hypersensitivity phenomena may occur, such as fever, rash, and eosinophilia [56]. About 15% of patients treated with NSAID presented significant elevations of liver-damaging enzymes, primarily alanine transaminase (ALT) and aspartate transaminase (AST), especially when administering Diclofenac and Sulindac [11]. Also, prostaglandins have an important role in female reproduction processes; it has been demonstrated by testing in mice the inhibition of COX-2 activity given by NSAID results in ovulation failure, fertilization, and implantation. Studies in animal models have also shown that these treatments modify the correct healing and union of fractures. Studies have not been conclusive since recovery depends on the type of wound, duration, and dose of the drug [57]. An increased risk of myocardial infarction has also been found in COX-2 inhibitors, presenting effects on blood pressure and nitric oxide production. Such is the case that ibuprofen interferes with the platelet effect and increases up to 35% risk of having myocardial infarction [58, 59].

On the other hand, the side effects of opioids include dry mouth [41], constipation, respiratory depression, nausea and urinary retention, motor impairment [60], as well as addiction, tolerance, and paradoxically hyperalgesia [42, 53]. Depression and respiratory disorders are a common and known treatment effect, caused by the activation of opioid receptors (*mu*, *kappa*, and *delta*) expressed in the brainstem respiratory centers [61]. In addition, opioids affect dopaminergic and adrenergic systems that can mediate reward and addiction pathways [62, 63]. Preclinical and clinical research has concluded that chronic opioid use alters endocrine functioning and food intake and increases body weight, which in turn is related to constipation and nausea [53, 64]. Excessive exposure to opioids may develop tolerance, through activation mediated by the NMDA receptor (N-methyl-D-aspartate) and an increase in pain sensitivity that manifests as hyperalgesia and/or allodynia in patients. NMDA receptor antagonists relieve tolerance and dependence on morphine [62, 63].

Due to their anticholinergic effect, TCAs can increase the risk of cardiovascular events and reduce secretions, so they are contraindicated in patients with kidney disease, urinary retention, glaucoma, or serious cardiovascular diseases. On the other hand, SSNIRs can cause hives, itching or rash, headache, restlessness, nausea, and dry mouth; they have also been associated with an increased risk of suicide in people suffering from major depression [44].

In synthesis, conventional therapies to treat different types of pain are not exempt from serious side effects and toxicity, particularly opioids, whose effects on the central and peripheral nervous system promote life-threatening respiratory depression, addiction, pruritus, nausea, and constipation [2]. This situation represents a serious health problem that has been increasing due to the practice of prescribing opioids for pain management [65].

7. Medicinal plants as potential treatment of pain: preclinical research

7.1 Animal models of pain

Animal experimentation has been a very important tool in elucidating the mechanism that underlies certain diseases [66] and contributes to the improvement of diagnostic and prophylactic procedures as well as the understanding of the etiology and pathogenicity of different diseases [67]. These animal models offer the advantage of their standardization, genetic, and environmental background [68].

Animal pain perception shows similarities to human pain; thus, animal models mimic the persistent pain found in the clinic, and thus, animal studies give an idea of certain aspects of human pain conditions and lead to better pain management in patients [69]. Most nociceptive assays involve a noxious stimulus that can be thermal, chemical, mechanical, or electrical to specific parts of the body, resulting in simple noxious behaviors that can be easily qualified [70]. On the other hand, neuropathic pain models involve an injury or disease that affects the somatosensory system and include spontaneous pain, painful hyperalgesia, or allodynia [71].

Although we define pain as a homogeneous sensory entity, it is important to emphasize the etiological distinction of pain, as it is one of the most important and studied to define the neurobiological mechanisms responsible and provide an idea of how different types of pain are generated [72].

Research into new treatments for pain relief and their mechanisms has justified the use of different animal models developed to better understand the progress of specific disease issues. However, one of the most important needs when implementing an experimental model is that it reflects the necessary clinical conditions, from inflammatory pain to chronic low back pain. Therefore, over time several animal models have been standardized that can evaluate different characteristics of pain. The **Table 3** shows the most important experimental pain models [1, 73–77].

7.2 Effects of medicinal plants on animal models of pain

Most often, pain is treated with allopathic or conventional pharmacological medicine, a vast pain conditions are complex to treat because of financial strains or adverse side effects. However, complementary and alternative medicine might be a novel solution because their great repertoire of techniques includes nonpharmacological remedies (massage, acupuncture, yoga, etc.) and the use of herbal medicine [5] to reduce opioid misuse, diminish avoidable costs, and improve health outcomes [78]. Therefore, herbal medicine is an important element of health systems in many developing and industrialized countries [79].

For the World Health Organization (WHO), "herbal medicines include herbs, herbal material, herbal preparations, and finished herbal products, which contain as active ingredients parts of plants, or other plant materials, or combinations of those elements" [80]. The popular use of medicinal plants in health care in many tropical and subtropical countries is widely described because of their enormous plant diversity. The consumption of medicinal plants has been important not only for the treatment of pain but also for treating diseases and metabolic disorders [81]. Therefore, the urge to gather more ethnobotanical and preclinical evidence to support the traditional uses of plants.

Nociceptive pain models		
Model	**Type of stimulus or injury**	**Natural metabolites evaluated**
Hot plate test Hargreaves test	Thermal	Organic compounds with possible antiharmful activity Substances with antiharmful properties, Flavonoids, Triterpenes, Carbohydrates, Phenols, Terpenoids, Coumarins, and Saponins, among others
Tail flick test	Thermal	
Tail immersion test	Thermal	
Paw/tail pressure test and Von Frey Randall-Selitto	Mechanical	
Electric stimulation of the tail	Electric	
Abdominal constriction test	Chemical	
Formalin test	Chemical	
Inflammatory pain models		
Model name	**Kind of stimulus or injury**	**Natural metabolites evaluated**
Capsaicin	Injection into skin, muscles, or joints	Phytochemical compounds with possible anti-inflammatory activity Polyphenols, Flavonoids, Quercetin, Phenolic compounds, Carotenoids, Quercetin, Catechin, Kaempferol, Epicatechins, Lupeol, Triterpenes, Phytosterols, Sterols, Lignans, Anthocyanins, and Alkaloids, among others.
Carrageenan	Injection into the leg, muscle, and joint	
Complete Freund Adjuvant (CFA)	Injection into the tail, leg, muscle, and joints	
Kaolin/carrageenan	Injection into knee or ankle joint	
Zymosan	Injection into knee or ankle joint	

Neuropathic pain models		
Model name	**Type of stimulus or injury**	**Natural metabolites evaluated**
Axotomy	Complete sciatic nerve transection	Opioids and tricyclic antidepressants, calcium antagonist (Verapamil, Nifedipine), sodium channel blockers (Lidocaine, Mexiletine, Tocainide), NMDA receptor antagonist (Dextromethorphan, Ketamine, Memantine), calcium N-channel blockers (Ziconotide), Antiepileptics (Gabapentin, Topiramate, Lamotrigine, Felbamate)
Chronic constriction injury	Four loose ligatures around sciatic nerve	
Partial sciatic nerve ligation (Seltzer Model)	Tight ligation of one-third to half of the sciatic nerve	
Spared nerve injury	Axotomy of tibial and common peroneal nerves	
Tibial and sural nerve transection	Axotomy of tibial and sural nerves	
Sciatic cryoneurolysis	Freezing of the sciatic nerve	
Sciatic inflammatory neuritis	Injection of zymosan, HMG, TNF-α around the sciatic nerve	
Laser-induced sciatic nerve injury	Radiation mediated reduction in blood supply to the sciatic nerve	
Excitotoxic spinal cord injury	Intraspinal injections of excitatory amino acids	
Spinal hemisection	Laminectomy of T11–T12 segments	
Diabetes-induced neuropathy	Persistent hyperglycemia-induced changes in the nerves	
Trigeminal neuralgia	Compression of trigeminal ganglion chronic constriction injury to the infraorbital nerve	
Orofacial pain	Injection of formalin, carrageenan into temporomandibular joints and maxilla	

Table 3.
Principal animal models of pain.

Several biological effects of extracts and purified compounds from herbal species have been tested *in vivo* and *in vitro* models. Extracts have shown antimicrobial, antiviral, and antimutagenic activity; cytotoxic activity for cancer cell lines and antinociceptive, anti-inflammatory activity; and antiatherogenic, antioxidant, and biocide for various food pests [82]. Based on the biological models of neuropathic pain, we can mention neuropathic pain induced by paclitaxel, chronic constriction injury, alcoholic neuropathy, streptozotocin-induced diabetic, partial sciatic nerve ligation, and model of sodium monoiodoacetate. Among the main secondary metabolites that have diminished pain are alkaloids, carotenes, flavonoids, phenols, and terpenes, among others [83]. Some species with analgesic profile and their metabolites are shown in **Table 4**.

The *Pterodon pubescens* (Benth) has been described as an analgesic. Phytochemistry studies have reported the presence of a high concentration of terpenes. The analgesic properties of *Pterodon pubescens* are attributed to these compounds [103]. An experimental study conducted in mice using the model of

Group of metabolite	Isolated metabolite	Plant containing the metabolite	Pharmacological effects	References
Alkaloid	Morphine Codeine Thebaine Papaverine	*Papaver somniferum* *Woodfordia fruticosa* *Peganum harmala*	Antinociceptive, anti-inflammatory, and antineuropathic	[84–86]
Flavonoid	Quercetin Rutin Kaempferol Luteolin Myricetin Apigenin	*Azadirachta indica* *Aloe vera* *Allium cepa* *Calamus scipionum* *Camellia sinensis* *Carica papaya* *Psidium guajava*	Peripheral neuropathy, anti-inflammatory, and antinociceptive	[87–90]
Carotene	β-carotene Lycopene	*Capsicum annuum* *Ginkgo biloba* *Solanum lycopersicum* *Daucus carota*	Acute or chronic pain: i.e. inhibiting the release of TNF-α and stimulating IL-10 production	[91, 92]
Phenol	Catechol Resorcinol Hydroquinone Phloroglucinol Vanillic acid Gallic acid	*Siegesbeckia orientalis* *Ageratum conyzoides* *Mikania cordifolia* *Moringa oleifera* *Plantago altissima* *Plantago lanceolata*	Antinociceptive and anti-inflammatory	[93–96]
Terpene	Thymoquinone Linalool Menthol Eugenol Fenchone Citronella	*Hyptis pectinata* *Hyptis fruticosa* *Erythrina velutina* *Aniba rosaeodora* *Mentha piperita* *Daphne aurantiaca*	Antinociceptive and anti-inflammatory	[97, 98]
Saponin	Digitonin Sarsasapogenin Dioscin	*Asparagus racemosus* *Tribulus terrestris*	Acute or chronic pain; antinociceptive, anti-inflammatory, and neuropathic	[99, 100]
Statins	Atorvastatin Lovastatin	*Trianthema portulacastrum*	Anti-nociceptive and anti-inflammatory	[101, 102]

Table 4.
Secondary metabolites with analgesic potential.

neuropathic pain induced by partial sciatic nerve ligation showed that the administration of ethanolic extract of *Pterodon pubescens*, at an oral dose of 300 mg/kg, was effective in exerting antinociceptive effects, revealing a possible mechanism of action associated with the significant bite suppression induced by kainate, glutamate, NMDA, and trans-ACPD. Also, the plant extract decreased the concentration of proinflammatory cytokines like TNF-α and IL-1β and the inhibition of channels of capsaicin (TRPV1) and cinnamaldehyde (TRPA1), respectively, without pharmacological tolerance. The most abundant metabolites extracted from these plants were sesquiterpenes and diterpenes, which suggest that these compounds are responsible for the therapeutic effect [104]. There is interest in the study of other plant species, including *Woodfordia fruticosa, Adhatoda vasica, Chenopodium ambrosioides, Viburnum cotinifolium, Vitex negundo, Peganum harmala,* and *Broussonetia papyrifera* because of the presence of effective alkaloids for pain treatment. The crude alkaloid extracts of all selected medicinal herbs were active at an oral dose of 1250 mg/kg of body weight in mice, where they reduced abdominal contractions caused by acetic acid and increased the latency time between the licks of the legs in both phases of pain (neuropathic and inflammatory) produced with formalin. In addition, the alkaloid-specific antinociceptive response was significantly in the naloxone model [86].

Another group of plants of pharmacological interest is the genus *Polygala* and the *Lamiaceae* family that have been widely used in pain therapy [105]. *Polygala molluginifolia* has shown important antinociceptive effects in mice. An experimental study showed that the hydroalcoholic extract of this plant, administered at a dose of 1000 mg/kg, exerted analgesic effects in a model of mechanical and thermal hyperalgesia to postoperative pain in mice. The mechanism of action of the experiment revealed that the effect of the natural product might be associated with a modulation of the TRPV1 and TRPA1 channels involved in nociceptive behavior and was demonstrated that *Polygala molluginifolia* has an antinociceptive potential without collateral effects like locomotor dysfunctions or sedation [106].

The phytochemistry of the species of the genus *Agastache* (Family *Lamiaceae*) is generally similar among them and consists of two classes of major metabolites: phenylpropanoids and terpenoids. The essential oils obtained from the family that has been identified more than 50% of estragole and volatile compounds such as methyl eugenol, pulegone, menthone, isomenthone, and spathulenol. The main nonvolatile metabolites are phenolic compounds, such as those derived from caffeic acid, especially rosmarinic acid, as well as several flavones and flavone glycosides such as acacetin, tilianin, agastachoside, and agastachin. Lignans, agastenol and agastinol, were also isolated, as well as terpenoids include oleanane type (maslinic acid, oleanolic acid, and β-amirin), ursane type (ursolic acid, corosolic acid, and α-amirin), typical plant sterols, and diterpenes (agastaquinone, agastol, and others) [82]. The plants of the *Lamiaceae* family are widely used as condiments, and some popular are oregano, thyme, and rosemary, but aromatic ones such as mint, basil, and sage are also part of this family [107].

About 250 species belong to the genus *Lippia* (Family *Verbenaceae*) and are distributed throughout Central and South America, as well as in the African continent. They are usually sold for the treatment of different types of pain, including stomach pain, abdominal pain, and headache, and are used as sedatives, anxiolytics, and anticonvulsants [108]. *Lippia alba, L. multiflora, L. gracilis, L. grata, L. origanoides, L. graveolens, L. geminata, L. origanoides,* and *L. adoensis* are the species that have reports worldwide on their effect on system disorders such as central nervous, pain, and inflammation [109].

Lippia origanoides commonly known in Mexico as "*oregano*" and *Lippia multiflora* also known in Africa are popularly used to control fever treat gastrointestinal disorders, enteritis, and cough. Composite leaves and flowers such as p-cymene, thymol, and carvacrol [110] were isolated from which the analgesic and antipyretic properties have been attributed, evaluated in mice and rats using carrageenan-induced hind paw as model of acute inflammation, and the analgesic effects were assayed by thermal, mechanical, and chemical models of antinociception, and this was correlated with an increase in glutathione and a decrease in nitric oxide and malondialdehyde, demonstrating a decrease in the levels of nitric acid and malonyl aldehyde process mediators such as inflammatory and pain [110]. A monoterpene called carvacrol has been isolated from oregano, which has shown antinociceptive effects. This metabolite was studied in an orofacial pain model and demonstrated that when administered at a dose of 20 mg/kg, it exerts antinociceptive effects in mice; however, this effect is punctuated more effectively if the metabolite is administered concomitantly with β-cyclodextrin [111]. Carvacrol/β-cyclodextrin has also been studied in cancer-induced pain models. Administered at a dose of 50 mg/kg, they exert antinociceptive effects in rodents that have tumors implanted in their hind paw [112]. An interesting fact about carvacrol is that its analgesic effects decrease when administered alone and increase when administered with cyclodextrin. On the other hand, carvacrol and p-cymene have an analgesic effect related to the decrease of pain mediators such as proinflammatory cytokines (IL-1, TNF, IL-4, TGF and IL-17) and anti-inflammatory (IL-10) [113, 114].

Hexane, ethyl acetate, and ethanol extracts from *Agastache mexicana subsp. xolocotziana* showed an antinociceptive effect in rats and mice. The ethyl acetate extract (containing significant amounts of ursolic acid) was the most active in the formalin-induced pain model, mainly in the inflammatory (second) phase; hexanic extract (present pulegonic and oleanolic acid) decreased thermal pain. The methanolic extract (rich in flavonoids such as acacetin and tilianin) was more active in the formalin model and in the acetic acid contortion model [82].

Rosemary plant has been assessed in Diabetes Mellitus cases of pain models. A study in rats showed that rosemary extract administration at 100, 150, and 200 mg/kg doses decreased hyperalgesia through the suppression of caspase-3. In this study, the neuroprotective effect of rosemary was also demonstrated, so that the authors suggested that the mechanisms of action might be involved in the inhibition of neuronal apoptosis [115].

The *Mentha spicata* plant, popularly known as garden mint, showed significant analgesic effects at the preclinical level. Phytochemical studies have revealed the presence of metabolites such as carvone, limonene, and menthol. Basil plant (*Ocimum basilicum*) has also shown analgesic effects combined with β-cyclodextrin. Studies have been conducted from basil essential oils, which are rich in monoterpenes. A study conducted in animal models of fibromyalgia showed that essential oils administered orally, at doses of 25, 50, and 100 mg/kg, significantly reduced mechanical hyperalgesia in mice [116, 117].

In addition to the plants described above, many others have presented significant effects in pain therapy in preclinical models associated with certain metabolites (see **Table 5**). Nevertheless, further molecular studies on secondary metabolites are needed, which allow to accurately indicate the mechanisms of action, and the effects can be compared with those analgesics already in the market. Further research is required to achieve analgesic effects at the lowest possible doses to significantly reduce the number of adverse reactions in organisms, particularly because the use of natural resources has become increasingly active in recent years because of the belief that natural products lack side effects [118]. Nevertheless, herbal therapy is risky because there are effects caused by plant metabolites that may vary depending on several external factors such as pollution, conservation processes, and the presence of pesticides, among others yet to be evaluated. As a result, the use of botanical medicine requires rigorous standardization processes that guarantee safety in its use [119]. The variety of soils and climates in such countries facilitates the growth of a wide range of plants. Nevertheless, the native people use plants empirically, which had led to the lack of standards in their use in terms of effectiveness, safety, and quality [120]. This idea has triggered the worldwide development of drugs used in plants, which lead to the phytomedicine trade worldwide [118].

Phytomedicine differs from synthetized chemical-pharmaceutical drugs in their components. A chemical-pharmaceutical drug is synthesized and designed in such a way we can have a pure compound or at least a small mixture of chemical molecules. Conversely, phytomedicine is plant extracts that contain numerous and not well-known compounds. As a result, the source of the plant material requires quality production and standardization of the extracts to guarantee the identification and purification of the compounds that target pain [121]. The increased popularity of herbal medicine worldwide had led to numerous reports that support its regulation. In some countries, regulations have been legally established in order

Plant	Potential active metabolite involved	Animal model used	Effects on pain	References
Cannabis sativa	Δ9-Tetrahydro-cannabinol Cannabidiol	Male and female mice in a chronic neuropathic sciatic nerve injury model	Reduce allodynia, hyperalgesia, and ultrasonic clicks	[123]
Papaver somniferum	Morphine	Male and female mice in a chronic neuropathic sciatic nerve injury model.	Reduce allodynia, hyperalgesia, and ultrasonic clicks but develop tolerance after 1 week	[123]
Urtica dioica, Urtica urens, and Urtica circularis	Phenolic compounds and hydroxy fatty acids	Anti-inflammatory *in vitro* COX-1 enzyme; Swiss mouse females in the formalin test and acetic acid-induced abdominal writhing test	Reduce the nociceptive response	[124, 125]
Verbesina persicifolia	Sesquiterpene-lactones (eudesman, cadinane, germacrane, and elemane)	TPA (12-O-tetradecanoylphorbol-13-acetate)-induced ear edema test	Anti-inflammatory activity	[126, 127]
Costus pictus, Costus spicatus	Flavonoids, flavonol glycosides, and polysaccharides	Male OF-1 mouse in formalin, acetic acid-induced abdominal writhing models; hot plate	Antinociceptive but not anti-inflammatory effect	[128, 129]
Valeriana officinalis	Sesquiterpene and iridoids	Orofacial formalin test	Reduce the nociceptive response	[130, 131]
Calotropis gigantea (L) R. Br.	Flavonoids, alkaloids, triterpenoids, steroids, saponins, phenols, and glycosides	Hot plate and acetic acid-induced abdominal writhing model	Decrease the number of paws licking and writhing	[132]
Curcuma longa L.	Alkaloids, flavonoids, saponins, and tannins Curcumin Demethoxy-curcumin Bisdemethoxy-curcumin	Acetic acid-induced induced abdominal writhing model. Tail flick test; tail immersion test	Reduce the number of writhing. Increase latency; reduce the tail withdrawal time	[133–135]
Gastrodia elata	4-Hidroxy-benzaldehyde 4-Hidroxybenzyl alcohol Benzyl alcohol Vanillin Vanillic acid	Carrageenan, acetic acid, arachidonic acid (AA)-induced paw edema and writhing models. Cyclooxygenase activity.	Analgesic and anti-inflammatory activity Inhibit the activity of COX-I/II	[136]
Spilanthes acmella, Acmella oleracea	Alkaloids, flavonoids, tannins, and carotenoids N-alkylamides Spilanthol	Formalin, capsaicin and cinnamaldehyde, carrageenan-induced paw edema models; hot plate and tail flick; traumatic sciatic nerve injury	Antinociceptive and anti-inflammatory effect; increase paw withdrawal latency and reduce mechanical allodynia	[137, 138]

Plant	Potential active metabolite involved	Animal model used	Effects on pain	References
Zingiber officinale	Alkaloid, flavonoids, and tannins	Hot plate, tail flick test; acetic acid-induced pain model	Antinociceptive effects against thermally and chemically stimulus	[139–141]
Salix alba	Alkaloids, tannins, polyphenolic salicin and glycosides 2-(hydroxymethyl)-phenyl-B-D-glucopyranoside Salicyl-alcohol	Formalin-induced paw edema model Enzymatic action of hyaluronidase	Inhibit the paw edema Inhibitory actions on biochemical pathways of arachidonic acid	[85, 142, 143]
Ammi majus	Furocoumarins and coumarins	Hot plate; formalin, carrageenan-hind paw edema models	Anti-inflammatory and antinociceptive; inhibition of the writhing number	[144, 145]
Arnica montana	Phenolic acids (caffeic, chlorogenic), flavonoids (quercetin, palutelin), sesquiterpene lactones (helenalin, dihydrohelenalin)	Hot plate; carrageenan, formalin-hind paw edema models; cytokines determination by ELISA	Inhibition of the licking, writhing, and biting response; decrease secretion of IL-6 and IL-8 proinflammatory cytokines	[146, 147]

Table 5.
Active metabolites in pain relief.

to safeguard public health, ensuring quality, efficiency, and safety. For instance, the European Union has one of the most complete regulatory systems for the use of herbal medicine [122]. Since the combination of both conventional and traditional herbal therapy has been poorly explored, it must be careful to avoid serious adverse reactions [81].

8. Final comments and conclusion

Pain is unpleasant sensory and emotional experience associated with actual or potential tissue damage, being one of the most persistent and disabling manifestations present in several conditions and diseases mentioned in this chapter, such as tissue injuries and bumps, postoperative surgery, cancer, diabetes, mood disorders, dementia, and schizophrenia, among others.

In this chapter, it was highlighted that the pain is continually reclassified due to its severity and complexity, coupled with the difficulty of describing it, despite the fact that there are currently more reliable and valid instruments. This activity is of great importance to improve the diagnosis and sure adequate therapeutic management.

Because pain is a global public health problem, there is a large class of drugs used for its treatment, such as opiates, tricyclic antidepressants, and antiepileptic drugs. As shown in this review, the prescription of this conventional painkiller depends on the type of pain, its duration, origin, and intensity. However, the side effects shown by these compounds hinder in many instances, their safe and effective use, particularly opioids, which could promote life-threatening respiratory depression, addiction, pruritus, nausea, and constipation. Therefore, new molecules are being sought with specific mechanisms of action that act from the genesis and maintenance of pain at different levels of the nervous system, for example, on the connexins, which would represent an outstanding advance.

On the other hand, in many countries, herbal medicine is used as a complementary or an alternative strategy to treat pain because it usually lowers costs, is more within reach of patients, and has an important cultural root. In this sense, species such as *Papaver somniferum, Pterodon pubescens, Capsicum annuum, Chenopodium ambrosioides, Polygala molluginifolia, Lippia alba, Agastache mexicana, Allium cepa, Moringa oleífera,* and *Hyptis pectinata,* among others described in this chapter are used due to their analgesics and anti-inflammatory properties. Secondary metabolites such as alkaloids, flavonoids, carotenes, terpenes, and other polyphenolic compounds seem to be responsible for the pharmacological effect reported, which has been demonstrated from the use of animal models, which show similar perception to chemical, thermal, electrical, and mechanical stimuli that can induce pain than in humans and that constitute one way to approach the study of new molecules or herbal extracts with analgesic activity.

Since the combination of both conventional and traditional phytotherapy has been poorly explored, this can often lead to harmful effects rather than improving pain treatment. Meanwhile, most analgesics and herbal products for pain treatment are accessible because they do not require a prescription for sale, their consumption has been exceeded, and self-medication has led to a major concern in several countries. Not regulated herbal therapies can trigger several conditions that may further compromise the patient's well-being. Currently, research on natural products includes the use of organic synthesis for improving natural product characteristics. Some research groups synthesize analogs of natural compounds and modify its activity to improve the effectiveness of the drug lead. Since the use of natural compounds might be risky because of the multiple active molecules present in plants, mimicking the targets that produce the desired effect, such as diminish pain, it is a useful alternative and avoids the burden of isolating molecules from natural resources. In this regard, it is possible to obtain a purified compound that can be tested. Molecular biology is a powerful tool to identify receptors and proteins, so a perspective in the pharmacological treatment of pain could be the development of further research in molecular biology for studying the targets of pain and therefore for designing specific molecules that can bind directly to pain receptors.

In conclusion, it is crucial that pharmaceutical, neuroscientists, and other healthcare professionals must be involved in well-designed preclinical trials to fully understand the effects of herbal medicines and phytopharmaceuticals and to study the molecular mechanisms and biological targets in which they operate. In terms of regulation, it would be important for organisms other than the Food and Drug Administration (FDA) in developing countries to establish the mechanisms such as to conduct all the preclinical trials before releasing a new drug.

Acknowledgements

Special thanks to the National Council of Science and Technology (CONACyT) for the postgraduate scholarships awarded to MFO-S (#635389), VDC-G (#927607), LSG-B (#782401), and the Program for Teacher Professional Development (PRODEP) for the financial support (#511–6/2019–2110,171/PPD-167).

Conflict of interest

The authors declare no conflict of interest.

Author details

Minerva Hernández Lozano[1*], Marcos Fernando Ocaña Sánchez[1,2], Rosa Virginia García Rodríguez[3], Van Dan Castro Gerónimo[2,3], Libna Sulem Gallardo Beatriz[3], Ibrahim Guillermo Castro Torres[4], María Gabriela Alcántara López[1], Julio César González Ortiz[5], Gabriela Josefina Mendoza Rangel[1] and Tania Monserrat Camacho Márquez[1]

1 Faculty of Biological Pharmaceutical Chemistry, University of Veracruz, Veracruz, Mexico

2 Biomedical Sciences, Biomedical Research Center, University of Veracruz, Xalapa, Veracruz, Mexico

3 Analytical Resolution Support Services Unit (SARA), University of Veracruz, Veracruz, Mexico

4 College of Sciences and Humanities, National Autonomous University of Mexico, Mexico City, Mexico

5 Department of Pain and Palliative Medicine, Institute for Social Security Services for State Employees (ISSSTE), Xalapa, Veracruz, Mexico

*Address all correspondence to: minehernandez@uv.mx

References

[1] Singh H, Bhushan S, Arora R, et al. Alternative treatment strategies for neuropathic pain: Role of Indian medicinal plants and compounds of plant origin—A review. Biomedicine and Pharmacotherapy. 2017;**92**:634-650

[2] Argoff CE. Topical analgesics in the management of acute and chronic pain. Mayo Clinic Proceedings. 2013;**88**:195-205

[3] Wehling M. Non-steroidal anti-inflammatory drug use in chronic pain conditions with special emphasis on the elderly and patients with relevant comorbidities: Management and mitigation of risks and adverse effects. European Journal of Clinical Pharmacology. 2014;**70**:1159-1172

[4] Randa H-D, Brunton LL, Goodman LS, editors. Goodman and Gilman's Manual of Pharmacology and Therapeutics. 2nd ed. New York, USA: McGraw-Hill; 2014

[5] Mishra S, Trikamji B, Togneri E. Complementary and alternative medicine in chronic neurological pain. Indian Journal of Pain. 2015;**29**:73-81

[6] Merskey H, Bogduk N. Classification of chronic pain. Descriptions of chronic pain syndromes and definitions of pain terms. Prepared by the international association for the study of pain, subcommittee on taxonomy. Pain Supplement. 1986;**3**:3

[7] Hanoch Kumar K, Elavarasi P. Definition of pain and classification of pain disorders. Journal of Advanced Clinical & Research Insights. 2016;**3**:87-90

[8] Li Z, Aninditha T, Griene B, et al. Burden of cancer pain in developing countries: A narrative literature review. ClinicoEconomics and Outcomes Research. 2018;**10**:675-691

[9] Sallum AMC, Garcia DM, Sanches M. Acute and chronic pain: A narrative review of the literature. Acta Paulista de Enfermagem. 2012;**25**: 150-154

[10] Guo Y, Wang Y, Sun Y, et al. A brain signature to differentiate acute and chronic pain in rats. Frontiers in Computational Neuroscience. **10**:1-11 [Epub ahead of print 28 April 2016]. DOI: 10.3389/fncom.2016.00041

[11] Crofford LJ. Use of NSAIDs in treating patients with arthritis. Arthritis Research and Therapy. **15**:1-10 [Epub ahead of print 24 July 2013]. DOI: 10.1186/ar4174

[12] Treede RD, Rief W, Barke A, et al. Chronic pain as a symptom or a disease: The IASP Classification of Chronic Pain for the International Classification of Diseases (ICD-11). Pain. 2019;**160**:19-27

[13] Freynhagen R, Parada HA, Calderon-Ospina CA, et al. Current understanding of the mixed pain concept: A brief narrative review. Current Medical Research and Opinion. 2019;**35**:1011-1018

[14] Fillingim RB, Loeser JD, Baron R, et al. Assessment of chronic pain: Domains, methods, and mechanisms. Journal of Pain. 2016;**17**:T10-T20

[15] Macfarlane GJ, Beasley M, Smith BH, et al. Can large surveys conducted on highly selected populations provide valid information on the epidemiology of common health conditions? An analysis of UK Biobank data on musculoskeletal pain. British Journal of Pain. 2015;**9**:203-212

[16] Gan TJ. Poorly controlled postoperative pain: Prevalence, consequences, and prevention. Journal of Pain Research. 2017;**10**:2287-2298

[17] Dahlhamer JM, Lucas J, Zelaya C, et al. Prevalence of chronic pain and high-impact chronic pain among adults—United States, 2016. Morbidity and Mortality Weekly Report. 2018;**67**: 1001-1006

[18] Pitcher MH, von Korff M, Bushnell MC, et al. Prevalence and profile of high-impact chronic pain in the United States. Journal of Pain. 2019;**20**:146-160

[19] Benjamin S, Barnes D, Berger S, et al. The relationship of chronic pain, mental illness and organic disorders. Pain. 1988;**32**:185-195

[20] Velly AM, Mohit S. Epidemiology of pain and relation to psychiatric disorders. Progress in Neuro-Psychopharmacology and Biological Psychiatry. 2018;**87**:159-167

[21] Stein MB, Steckler T. Behavioral neurobiology of anxiety and its treatment. Preface. Current Topics in Behavioral Neurosciences. 2010;**2**:v-vii

[22] Babel P. The influence of state and trait anxiety on the memory of pain. Pain Medicine (United States). 2017;**18**:2340-2349

[23] Bernstein MT, Mackenzie CS, Sareen J, et al. Examining the cross-sectional and longitudinal effects of anxiety sensitivity on indicators of disease severity among patients with inflammatory arthritis. Journal of Anxiety Disorders. **67**:1-8 [Epub ahead of print 01 October 2019]. DOI: 10.1016/j.janxdis.2019.102117

[24] Uebelacker LA, van Noppen D, Tremont G, et al. A pilot study assessing acceptability and feasibility of hatha yoga for chronic pain in people receiving opioid agonist therapy for opioid use disorder. Journal of Substance Abuse Treatment. 2019;**105**:19-27

[25] Woo AK. Depression and Anxiety in Pain. Reviews in Pain. 2010;**4**:8-12

[26] Smith K. Mental health: A world of depression. Nature. 2014;**515**:181

[27] Bair MJ, Robinson RL, Katon W, et al. Depression and pain comorbidity: A literature review. Archives of Internal Medicine. 2003;**163**:2433-2445

[28] Sacuiu SF. Dementias. Handbook of Clinical Neurology. 2016;**138**:123-151

[29] Ferencz B, Gerritsen L. Genetics and underlying pathology of dementia. Neuropsychology Review. 2015;**25**:113-124

[30] Gagliese L, Gauthier LR, Narain N, et al. Pain, aging and dementia: Towards a biopsychosocial model. Progress in Neuro-Psychopharmacology and Biological Psychiatry. 2018;**87**:207-215

[31] Herr K, Zwakhalen S, Swafford K. Observation of pain in dementia. Current Alzheimer Research. 2016;**14**: 486-500

[32] Tomasik J, Rahmoune H, Guest PC, et al. Neuroimmune biomarkers in schizophrenia. Schizophrenia Research. 2016;**176**:3-13

[33] Soria V, Uribe J, Salvat-Pujol N, et al. Psychoneuroimmunology of mental disorders. Revista de Psiquiatria y Salud Mental. 2018;**11**:115-124

[34] Antioch I, Ciobica A, Paulet M, et al. Pain manifestations in schizophrenia—Clinical and experimental aspects in human patients and animal models. Psychiatria Danubina. 2015;**27**:142-152

[35] Flower RJ. Drugs which inhibit prostaglandin biosynthesis. Pharmacological Reviews. 1974;**26**:33-67

[36] Vane JR, Botting RM. Mechanism of action of nonsteroidal anti-inflammatory drugs. American Journal of Medicine. 1998 [Epub ahead of print 30 March 1998]. DOI: 10.1016/S0002-9343(97)00203-9

[37] Hodkinson DJ, Khawaja N, O'Daly O, et al. Cerebral analgesic response to nonsteroidal anti-inflammatory drug ibuprofen. Pain. 2015;**156**:1301-1310

[38] Cashman JN. The mechanisms of action of NSAIDs in analgesia. Drugs. 1996;**52**:13-23. https://doi.org/10.2165/00003495-199600525-00004

[39] Girard P, Verniers D, Coppé MC, et al. Nefopam and ketoprofen synergy in rodent models of antinociception. European Journal of Pharmacology. 2008;**584**:263-271

[40] Vargas CG, Miranda HF, Sierralta F, et al. Pharmacological interaction between NSAIDS with clomipramine and risperidone in mice visceral pain. Drug Development Research. 2019;**80**:471-474

[41] Khademi H, Kamangar F, Brennan P, et al. Opioid therapy and its side effects: A review. Archives of Iranian Medicine. 2016;**19**:870-876

[42] Ribeiro MMB, Santos SS, Sousa DSC, et al. Side-effects of analgesic kyotorphin derivatives: Advantages over clinical opioid drugs. Amino Acids. 2013;**45**: 171-178

[43] Xu L, Zhang Y, Huang Y. Advances in the treatment of neuropathic pain. In: Advances in Experimental Medicine and Biology. New York: Springer LLC; 2016. pp. 117-129

[44] Yan YY, Li CY, Zhou L, et al. Research progress of mechanisms and drug therapy for neuropathic pain. Life Sciences. 2017;**190**:68-77

[45] Mathieson S, Maher CG, McLachlan AJ, et al. Trial of pregabalin for acute and chronic sciatica. New England Journal of Medicine. 2017;**376**:1111-1120

[46] Zakrzewska JM, Linskey ME. Trigeminal neuralgia. BMJ Clinical Evidence. 2014:1-3 [Epub ahead of print 06 October 2014]. DOI: 10.1097/00005053-192,304,000-00042

[47] Cruccu G. Trigeminal neuralgia. Continuum Lifelong Learning in Neurology. 2017;**23**:396-420

[48] Xu B, Descalzi G, Ye HR, et al. Translational investigation and treatment of neuropathic pain. Molecular Pain. **8**:1-8 [Epub ahead of print 09 March 2012]. DOI: 10.1186/1744-8069-8-15

[49] Alcántara-Montero A. Desvenlafaxina y dolor neuropático: Beneficios clínicos adicionales de un inhibidor de la recaptación de serotonina-noradrenalina de segunda generación. Revista de Neurologia. 2017;**64**:219-226

[50] Kim W, Chung Y, Choi S, et al. Duloxetine protects against oxaliplatin-induced neuropathic pain and spinal neuron hyperexcitability in rodents. International Journal of Molecular Sciences. **18**:1-10 [Epub ahead of print 05 December 2017]. DOI: 10.3390/ijms18122626

[51] Morioka N, Nakamura Y, Zhang FF, et al. Role of connexins in chronic pain and their potential as therapeutic targets for next-generation analgesics. Biological and Pharmaceutical Bulletin. 2019;**42**:857-866

[52] Paracetamol: Uses, Dosage & Side Effects. Available from: Drugs.com, https://www.drugs.com/paracetamol.html [Accessed: 15 December 2019]

[53] Jirkof P. Side effects of pain and analgesia in animal experimentation. Lab Animal. 2017;**46**:123-128

[54] Domiati S, El-Mallah A, Ghoneim A, et al. Evaluation of anti-inflammatory, analgesic activities, and side effects of some pyrazole derivatives. Inflammopharmacology. 2016;**24**:163-172

[55] Aronson JK. Meyler's Side Effects of Analgesics and Anti-inflammatory Drugs. California, USA: Elsevier Science; 2010

[56] Moreno-Brea M. Aspirin tolerability. Revista de la Sociedad Española del Dolor. 2005;**12**:357-372

[57] Parker JM, Austin J, Wilkerson J, et al. Effects of multimodal analgesia on the success of mouse embryo transfer surgery. Journal of the American Association for Laboratory Animal Science. 2011;**50**:466-470

[58] Trelle S, Reichenbach S, Wandel S, et al. Cardiovascular safety of non-steroidal anti-inflammatory drugs: Network meta-analysis. British Medical Journal. 2011;**342**:154

[59] García Rodríguez LA, Tacconelli S, Patrignani P. Role of dose potency in the prediction of risk of myocardial infarction associated with nonsteroidal anti-inflammatory drugs in the general population. Journal of the American College of Cardiology. 2008;**52**:1628-1636

[60] Jamison RN, Dorado K, Mei A, et al. Influence of opioid-related side effects on disability, mood, and opioid misuse risk among patients with chronic pain in primary care. Pain Reports. **2**:1-7 [Epub ahead of print 01 March 2017]. DOI: 10.1097/PR9.0000000000000589

[61] van der Schier R, Roozekrans M, van Velzen M, et al. Opioid-induced respiratory depression: Reversal by non-opioid drugs. F1000Prime Reports. **6**:1-8 [Epub ahead of print 2014]. DOI: 10.12703/P6-79

[62] Tabatabai SM, Dashti S, Doosti F, et al. Phytotherapy of opioid dependence and withdrawal syndrome: A review. Phytotherapy Research. 2014;**28**:811-830

[63] Cheatle MD. Prescription opioid misuse, abuse, morbidity, and mortality: Balancing effective pain management and safety. Pain Medicine (United States). 2015;**16**:S3-S8

[64] Webster L, Camilleri M, Finn A. Opioid-induced constipation: Rationale for the role of norbuprenorphine in buprenorphine-treated individuals. Substance Abuse and Rehabilitation. 2016;**81**:81-86

[65] Carter GT, Duong V, Ho S, et al. Side effects of commonly prescribed analgesic medications. Physical Medicine and Rehabilitation Clinics of North America. 2014;**25**:457-470

[66] Bart van der Worp H, Howells DW, Sena ES, et al. Can animal models of disease reliably inform human studies? PLoS Medicine. 2010;**7**:1-8

[67] Deuis JR, Dvorakova LS, Vetter I. Methods used to evaluate pain behaviors in rodents. Frontiers in Molecular Neuroscience. **10**:1-17 [Epub ahead of print 06 September 2017]. DOI: 10.3389/fnmol.2017.00284

[68] Mogil JS, Davis KD, Derbyshire SW. The necessity of animal models in pain research. Pain. 2010;**151**:12-17

[69] Ma C, Zhang J-M. Animal Models of Pain. Totowa, New Jersey: Humana Press; pp. 1-21 [Epub ahead of print 2011]. DOI: 10.1016/s0896-6273(02)00780-8

[70] Mogil JS. Animal models of pain: Progress and challenges. Nature Reviews Neuroscience. 2009;**10**:283-294

[71] Jensen TS, Baron R, Haanpää M, et al. A new definition of neuropathic pain. Pain. 2011;**152**:2204-2205

[72] Treede RD, Rief W, Barke A, et al. A classification of chronic pain for ICD-11. Pain. 2015;**156**:1003-1007

[73] Colloca L, Ludman T, Bouhassira D, et al. Neuropathic pain. Nature Reviews Disease Primers. **3**:1-19 [Epub ahead of

print 16 February 2017]. DOI: 10.1038/nrdp.2017.2

[74] Burma NE, Leduc-Pessah H, Fan CY, et al. Animal models of chronic pain: Advances and challenges for clinical translation. Journal of Neuroscience Research. 2017;**95**:1242-1256

[75] Barrett JE. The pain of pain: Challenges of animal behavior models. European Journal of Pharmacology. 2015;**753**:183-190

[76] Gregory NS, Harris AL, Robinson CR, et al. An overview of animal models of pain: Disease models and outcome measures. Journal of Pain. 2013;**14**:1255-1269

[77] Barrot M. Tests and models of nociception and pain in rodents. Neuroscience. 2012;**211**:39-50

[78] Hooten M, Thorson D, Bianco J, et al. Pain: Assessment, non-opioid treatment approaches and opioid management 2017 . Available from: www.icsi.org [Accessed: 15 December 2019]

[79] Šantić Ž, Pravdić N, Bevanda M, et al. The historical use of medicinal plants in traditional and scientific medicine. Psychiatria Danubina. 2017;**29**:787-792

[80] World Health Organization (WHO). General Guidelines for Methodologies on Research and Evaluation of Traditional Medicine. London, UK: Stationery Office Books. pp. 1-80

[81] Heinrich M. Ethnopharmacology: Quo vadis? Challenges for the future. Brazilian Journal of Pharmacognosy. 2014;**24**:99-102

[82] Zielińska S, Matkowski A. Phytochemistry and bioactivity of aromatic and medicinal plants from the genus Agastache (Lamiaceae). Phytochemistry Reviews. 2014;**13**: 391-416

[83] Quintans JSS, Antoniolli ÂR, Almeida JRGS, et al. Natural products evaluated in neuropathic pain models—A systematic review. Basic and Clinical Pharmacology and Toxicology. 2014;**114**:442-450

[84] Sayhan H, Beyaz SG, Çeliktaş A. The local anesthetic and pain relief activity of alkaloids. In: Alkaloids—Alternatives in Synthesis, Modification and Application. Rijeka: InTechOpen. 2017 [Epub ahead of print 12 July 2017]. DOI: 10.5772/intechopen.69847

[85] McCurdy CR, Scully SS. Analgesic substances derived from natural products (natureceuticals). Life Sciences. 2005;**78**:476-484. https://doi.org/10.1016/j.lfs.2005.09.006

[86] Shoaib M, Shah SWA, Ali N, et al. Scientific investigation of crude alkaloids from medicinal plants for the management of pain. BMC Complementary and Alternative Medicine. **16**:1-8 [Epub ahead of print 13 June 2016]. DOI: 10.1186/s12906-016-1157-2

[87] Narenjkar J, Roghani M, Alambeygi H, et al. The effect of the flavonoid quercetin on pain sensation in diabetic rats. Basic and Clinical Neuroscience. 2011;**2**:51-57

[88] Sultana B, Anwar F. Flavonols (kaempeferol, quercetin, myricetin) contents of selected fruits, vegetables and medicinal plants. Food Chemistry. 2008;**108**:879-884

[89] Miean KH, Mohamed S. Flavonoid (myricetin, quercetin, kaempferol, luteolin, and apigenin) content of edible tropical plants. Journal of Agricultural and Food Chemistry. 2001;**49**:3106-3112

[90] Azevedo MI, Pereira AF, Nogueira RB, et al. The antioxidant effects of the flavonoids rutin and quercetin inhibit oxaliplatin-induced chronic painful peripheral neuropathy.

Molecular Pain. **9**:1-14 [Epub ahead of print 23 October 2013]. DOI: 10.1186/1744-8069-9-53

[91] Hazewindus M, Haenen GRMM, Weseler AR, et al. The anti-inflammatory effect of lycopene complements the antioxidant action of ascorbic acid and α-tocopherol. Food Chemistry. 2012;**132**:954-958

[92] Kuhad A, Sharma S, Chopra K. Lycopene attenuates thermal hyperalgesia in a diabetic mouse model of neuropathic pain. European Journal of Pain. 2008;**12**:624-632

[93] Beara IN, Lesjak MM, Orčić DZ, et al. Comparative analysis of phenolic profile, antioxidant, anti-inflammatory and cytotoxic activity of two closely-related Plantain species: *Plantago altissima* L. and *Plantago lanceolata* L. LWT—Food Science and Technology. 2012;**47**:64-70

[94] Cheenpracha S, Park EJ, Yoshida WY, et al. Potential anti-inflammatory phenolic glycosides from the medicinal plant *Moringa oleifera* fruits. Bioorganic and Medicinal Chemistry. 2010;**18**:6598-6602

[95] Dewan SMR, Amin MN, Adnan T, et al. Investigation of analgesic potential and in vitro antioxidant activity of two plants of Asteraceae family growing in Bangladesh. Journal of Pharmacy Research. 2013;**6**:599-603

[96] Tuberoso CIG, Orrù CD. Phenolic compounds in food. In: Koeffer EN, editor. Progress in Food Chemistry. New York, USA: Nova Science Publishers, Inc.; 2008. pp. 1-45

[97] Liang S, Shen Y-H, Feng Y, et al. Terpenoids from *Daphne aurantiaca* and their potential anti-inflammatory activity. Journal of Natural Products. 2010;**73**:532-535

[98] de Sousa DP. Analgesic-like activity of essential oils constituents. Molecules. 2011;**16**:2233-2252

[99] Chawla A, Chawla P, Mangalesh, Roy RC. *Asparagus racemosus* (Willd): Biological activities & its active principles. Indo Global Journal of Pharmaceutical Sciences. 2011;**1**(2):113

[100] Gautam M, Ramanathan M. Saponins of *Tribulus terrestris* attenuated neuropathic pain induced with vincristine through central and peripheral mechanism. Inflammopharmacology. 2019;**27**:761-772

[101] Garcia GG, Miranda HF, Noriega V, et al. Antinociception induced by atorvastatin in different pain models. Pharmacology Biochemistry and Behavior. 2011;**100**:125-129

[102] Sunder AS, Reddy ARN, Kiran G, et al. Antihyperlipidemic and antioxidant activity of methanolic extract of *Trianthema portulacastrum* in rats fed a high-fat diet. Journal of Herbs, Spices and Medicinal Plants. 2010;**16**:193-202

[103] Forouzanfar F, Hosseinzadeh H. Medicinal herbs in the treatment of neuropathic pain: A review. Iranian Journal of Basic Medical Sciences. 2018;**21**:347-358

[104] Nucci-Martins C, Martins DF, Nascimento LF, et al. Ameliorative potential of standardized fruit extract of *Pterodon pubescens* Benth on neuropathic pain in mice: Evidence for the mechanisms of action. Journal of Ethnopharmacology. 2015;**175**:273-286

[105] Uritu CM, Mihai CT, Stanciu GD, et al. Medicinal plants of the family Lamiaceae in pain therapy: A review. Pain Research and Management. 2018:1-45 [Epub ahead of print 2018]. DOI. DOI: 10.1155/2018/7801543

[106] Nucci-Martins C, Nascimento LF, Venzke D, et al. Antinociceptive effect of hydroalcoholic extract and isoflavone isolated from Polygala molluginifolia in mice: Evidence for the involvement of opioid receptors and TRPV1 and TRPA1

channels. Phytomedicine. 2016;**23**: 429-440

[107] Bekut M, Brkić S, Kladar N, et al. Potential of selected Lamiaceae plants in anti(retro)viral therapy. Pharmacological Research. 2018;**133**:301-314

[108] Pascual ME, Slowing K, Carretero E, et al. Lippia: Traditional uses, chemistry and pharmacology: A review. Journal of Ethnopharmacology. 2001;**76**:201-214

[109] Siqueira-Lima PS, Passos FRS, Lucchese AM, et al. Central nervous system and analgesic profiles of Lippia genus. Brazilian Journal of Pharmacognosy. 2019;**29**:125-135

[110] Abena AA, Diatewa M, Gakosso G, et al. Analgesic, antipyretic and anti-inflammatory effects of essential oil of *Lippia multiflora*. Fitoterapia. 2003;**74**: 231-236

[111] Silva JC, Almeida JRGS, Quintans JSS, et al. Enhancement of orofacial antinociceptive effect of carvacrol, a monoterpene present in oregano and thyme oils, by β-cyclodextrin inclusion complex in mice. Biomedicine and Pharmacotherapy. 2016;**84**:454-461

[112] Guimarães AG, Oliveira MA, Alves RDS, et al. Encapsulation of carvacrol, a monoterpene present in the essential oil of oregano, with β-cyclodextrin, improves the pharmacological response on cancer pain experimental protocols. Chemico-Biological Interactions. 2015;**227**:69-76

[113] de Santana MF, Guimarães AG, Chaves DO, et al. The anti-hyperalgesic and anti-inflammatory profiles of p-cymene: Evidence for the involvement of opioid system and cytokines. Pharmaceutical Biology. 2015;**53**:1583-1590

[114] Kianmehr M, Rezaei A, Boskabady MH. Effect of carvacrol on various cytokines genes expression in splenocytes of asthmatic mice. Iranian Journal of Basic Medical Sciences. 2016;**19**:402-410

[115] Rasoulian B, Hajializadeh Z, Esmaeili-Mahani S, et al. Neuroprotective and antinociceptive effects of rosemary (*Rosmarinus officinalis* L.) extract in rats with painful diabetic neuropathy. Journal of Physiological Sciences. 2019;**69**:57-64

[116] Mahboubi M. Mentha spicata as natural analgesia for treatment of pain in osteoarthritis patients. Complementary Therapies in Clinical Practice. 2017;**26**:1-4

[117] Nascimento SS, Araújo AAS, Brito RG, et al. Cyclodextrin-complexed *Ocimum basilicum* leaves essential oil increases fos protein expression in the central nervous system and produce an antihyperalgesic effect in animal models for fibromyalgia. International Journal of Molecular Sciences. 2015;**16**:547-563

[118] Atul Bhattaram V, Graefe U, Kohlert C, et al. Pharmacokinetics and bioavailability of herbal medicinal products. Phytomedicine. 2002;**9**:1-33

[119] Schlaepfer L, Mendoza-Espinoza JA. Medicinal plants as potential agents against cancer, relevance for Mexico. Revista Mexicana de Ciencias Farmaceuticas. 2016;**4**:26-34

[120] Karunamoorthi K, Jegajeevanram K, Vijayalakshmi J, et al. Traditional medicinal plants. Journal of Evidence-Based Complementary & Alternative Medicine. 2013;**18**:67-74

[121] Allemann C, Herren D, Mathys BK. Quality requirements of approved herbal medicinal products. Therapeutische Umschau. 2002;**59**:267-273

[122] Qu L, Zou W, Wang YT, et al. European regulation model for herbal medicine: The assessment of the EU monograph and the safety and efficacy

evaluation in marketing authorization or registration in Member States. Phytomedicine. 2018;**42**:219-225

[123] Abraham AD, Leung EJY, Wong BA, Rivera ZMG, Kruse LC, Clark JJ, et al. Orally consumed cannabinoids provide long-lasting relief of allodynia in a mouse model of chronic neuropathic pain. Neuropsychopharmacology. 2019:1-10. https://doi.org/10.1038/s41386-019-0585-3

[124] Farag MA, Weigend M, Luebert F, et al. Phytochemical, phylogenetic, and anti-inflammatory evaluation of 43 Urtica accessions (stinging nettle) based on UPLC-Q-TOF-MS metabolomic profiles. Phytochemistry. 2013;**96**:170-183

[125] Marrassini C, Acevedo C, Miño J, et al. Evaluation of antinociceptive, antinflammatory activities and phytochemical analysis of aerial parts of Urtica urens L. Phytotherapy Research. 2010;**24**:1807-1812

[126] Jakupovic J, Ellmauerer E, Jia Y. Further eudesmane derivatives from Verbesina species. Planta Medica. 1987;**53**:39-42

[127] Dalla Via L, Mejia M, García-Argáez AN, et al. Anti-inflammatory and antiproliferative evaluation of 4β-cinnamoyloxy,1β,3α-dihydroxyeudesm-7,8-ene from Verbesina persicifolia and derivatives. Bioorganic and Medicinal Chemistry. 2015;**23**:5816-5828

[128] Morón Rodríguez F, Victoria Amador MdC, Morejón Rodríguez Z, et al. Tamizaje fitoquímico, actividad analgésica y antiinflamatoria de decocción de Costus pictus D. Don decoction [Phytochemical screening, analgesic and antiinflammatory properties of Costus pictus D. Don.]. Revista Cubana de Plantas Medicinales. 2008;**13**. Available from: http://scielo.sld.cu/scielo.php?script=sci_arttext&pid=S1028-47962008000400013 [Accessed: 15 December 2019]

[129] Quintans Júnior LJ, Santana MT, Melo MS, et al. Antinociceptive and anti-inflammatory effects of *Costus spicatus* in experimental animals. Pharmaceutical Biology. 2010;**48**:1097-1102

[130] Nowacki LC, Worfel PR, Martins PFA, et al. Analgesic effect of *Hypericum perforatum*, *Valeriana officinalis* and *Piper methysticum* for orofacial pain. Brazilian Journal of Oral Sciences. 2015;**14**:60-65

[131] Torkamani MRD, Abbaspour N, Jafari M, et al. Elicitation of valerenic acid in the hairy root cultures of *Valeriana officinalis* L. (Valerianaceae). Tropical Journal of Pharmaceutical Research. 2014;**13**:943-949

[132] Pathak AK, Argal A. Analgesic activity of *Calotropis gigantea* flower. Fitoterapia. 2007;**78**:40-42

[133] Neha S, Ranvir GD, Jangade CR. Analgesic and antipyretic activities of Curcuma longa rhizome extracts in Wister Rats. 2009. Available from: www.veterinaryworld.org [Accessed: 15 December 2019]

[134] Hasan MN, Ferdoushi A, Ara N, et al. Preliminary phytochemical screening, toxicity, antihyperglycemic and analgesic activity studies with Curcuma longa leaves. World Journal of Pharmacy and Pharmaceutical Sciences. 2014;**3**:81-91

[135] John S, Nikhil S, Yaswanth J, et al. Analgesic property of different extracts of *Curcuma longa* (Linn.): An experimental study in animals. Journal of Natural Remedies. 2009;**9**:116-120

[136] Ji YL, Young WJ, Hyo SK, et al. Anti-inflammatory action of phenolic

compounds from Gastrodia elata root. Archives of Pharmacal Research. 2006;**29**:849-858

[137] Nomura ECO, Rodrigues MRA, da Silva CF, et al. Antinociceptive effects of ethanolic extract from the flowers of *Acmella oleracea* (L.) R.K. Jansen in mice. Journal of Ethnopharmacology. 2013;**150**:583-589

[138] Chakraborty A, Devi RKB, Rita S, et al. Preliminary studies on antiinflammatory and analgesic activities of *Spilanthes acmella* in experimental animal models. Indian Journal of Pharmacology. 2004;**36**:148-150

[139] Ojewole JAO. Analgesic, antiinflammatory and hypoglycaemic effects of ethanol extract of *Zingiber officinale* (Roscoe) rhizomes (Zingiberaceae) in mice and rats. Phytotherapy Research. 2006;**20**:764-772

[140] Sepahvand R, Esmaeili-Mahani S, Arzi A, et al. Ginger (*Zingiber officinale* Roscoe) elicits antinociceptive properties and potentiates morphine-induced analgesia in the rat radiant heat tail-flick test. Journal of Medicinal Food. 2010;**13**:1397-1401

[141] Otunola GA, Oloyede OB, Oladiji AT, et al. Comparative analysis of the chemical composition of three spices—*Allium sativum* L. *Zingiber officinale* Rosc. and *Capsicum frutescens* L. commonly consumed in Nigeria. African Journal of Biotechnology. 2010;**9**:6927-6931

[142] Gyawali R, Bhattarai P, Dhakal S, et al. Analgesic and anti-inflammatory properties of *Salix alba* Linn and *Calotropis procera* (Aiton) Dryand. 2013. Available from: www.ijpba.info [Accessed: 15 December 2019]

[143] Bodîrlău R, Spiridon I, Teacâ CA, et al. Anti-inflammatory constituents from different plant species. Environmental Engineering and Management Journal. 2009;**8**(4):785-792

[144] Koriem KMM, Asaad GF, Megahed HA, et al. Evaluation of the antihyperlipidemic, anti-inflammatory, analgesic, and antipyretic activities of ethanolic extract of *Ammi majus* seeds in albino rats and mice. International Journal of Toxicology. 2012;**31**:294-300

[145] Mutlag SH. Dose dependent anti-inflammatory effect of *Ammi majus* alcoholic extract in rat: Chronic study. Iraqi Journal of Pharmaceutical Sciences. 2012;**21**:82-86

[146] Ahmad M, Saeed F, Mehjabeen, et al. Neuro-pharmacological and analgesic effects of *Arnica montana* extract. International Journal of Pharmacy and Pharmaceutical Sciences. 2013;**5**:590-593

[147] Gaspar A, Craciunescu O, Trif M, Moisei M, Moldovan L. Antioxidant and anti-inflammatory properties of active compounds from *Arnica montana* L. Romanian Biotechnological Letters. 2014;**9**(3):9353-9365

Chapter 5

Neuropharmacology of Secondary Metabolites from Plants with Anxiolytic and Antidepressant Properties

Rosa Isela García-Ríos, Armando Mora-Pérez, Ana Raquel Ramos-Molina and Cesar Soria-Fregozo

Abstract

Depression and anxiety currently rank as the second and fifth most common causes worldwide of years lived with disability-a reality that has intensified the search for new treatments. There are many studies of herbal extracts and secondary metabolites from plants used in traditional medicine due to their antidepressant and anxiolytic properties. Clinical and preclinical studies about some of the mechanisms of action of metabolites like alkaloids, terpenes, flavonoids, and sterols, among others, have documented effects similar to those produced by clinically effective drugs. These metabolites have shown anxiolytic and antidepressant effects in various experimental models of anxiety by interacting with γ-aminobutyric acid subtype A receptors ($GABA_A$-receptors) and by stimulating the serotonergic, noradrenergic, and dopaminergic neurotransmitter systems. These pharmacological effects can be attributed to plant metabolites that share structural similarities with monoamines, which allow them to bind to receptors. The objective of this chapter is to summarize the various mechanisms of action that have been identified in secondary metabolites with anxiolytic and antidepressant properties. Terpenes, alkaloids, flavonoids, and sterols can interact at different levels of the neurotransmission systems involved in the neurobiology of anxiety and depression, suggesting their potential for treating these mental illnesses.

Keywords: antidepressant, anxiolytic, active metabolites, plant extracts, herbal medicines

1. Introduction

According to the Global Burden of Disease, depression and anxiety are currently the second and fifth most common causes worldwide of years lived with disability in both sexes in the age range of 15–49 years [1]. In 2015, 4.4% (322 million people) of the world's population suffered from depressive disorders, while 3.6% (264 million) were affected by anxiety [2]. In that year, the World Health Organization (WHO) estimated that by 2020 depression would be the second leading cause of disability; thus, its prediction has been confirmed. Depression is characterized by persistent sadness and a loss of interest in activities that an individual normally enjoys, accompanied by periods of at least 2 weeks marked by the inability to perform everyday activities [2]. Anxiety, in turn, is defined as an emotion expressed in response to stressful, dangerous, or unfamiliar situations, or some unidentified factor, that is, the feeling of unease, distress, or dread that one feels in the face of a significant event. A certain level of anxiety is necessary to keep us alert and aware, but for those who suffer from anxiety disorders, it can be totally debilitating [3]. Current pharmacological treatments for depressive disorders are mainly based on selective serotonin reuptake inhibitors (SSRIs), serotonin (5-HT) and noradrenaline (NE) reuptake inhibitors (SNRIs), and monoamine oxidase inhibitors (MAOIs), all of which act by increasing short-term levels of neurotransmitters in the brain. One consequence of treatment is the desensitization of receptors, for example, 5-HT_{1A}, with a downregulation of autoreceptors, but no changes in the postsynaptic receptors, which leads to the recovery of neuronal activity in the long term [4]. These changes are associated with the long latency to the onset of antidepressant effects. However, up to 70% of depressed patients have residual symptoms [5], and few options exist for transitioning treatment-resistant sufferers to alternative therapies that operate through distinct mechanisms [6]. It is important to note that conventional antidepressants produce significant side effects, such as nausea and vomiting, insomnia, agitation, fatigue, sedation, sexual dysfunction, headaches, and weight gain, which contribute to poor patient compliance and, in some cases, abandonment of treatment [7]. This occurs under such anxiolytic treatments as benzodiazepine (a $GABA_A$ receptor agonist) and SSRIs [8] and is the main cause of the increasing demand for alternative medicines, such as medicinal plants, to alleviate the symptoms of these psychiatric disorders. However, reports of adverse reactions to products of this kind have increased [9], leading WHO to publish the document, "The WHO's traditional medicine strategy: 2014-2023", which outlines a global approach to fomenting the appropriate integration, regulation, and supervision of natural substances. This paper will be useful in countries seeking to develop a proactive policy toward this important and expanding area of health care and will contribute to the use of herbal medicines of proven quality, safety, and efficacy, providing quality medical care to all people [10]. Recent decades have witnessed efforts to gather scientific evidence that validates the efficacy of plants commonly used for their antidepressant and anxiolytic properties [11], but research has been insufficient because of the wide range of plants available worldwide. We lack solid scientific data on the neurochemical pathways and mechanisms of action of medicinal plants or their active metabolites because few clinical studies have addressed these issues. Also, reports of adverse reactions to medicinal plants [9] may reflect the broad variety of active metabolites they contain, thus highlighting the need for preclinical and clinical studies that evaluate the possible biological activity of compounds isolated from plants or standardized crude extracts, their mechanisms of action, and possible toxicity.

Fajemiroye et al. [12] proposed a hypothetical model for identifying medicinal plant extracts and phytoconstituents with anxiolytic and/or antidepressant properties that is currently used by most researchers: *(i) select medicinal plants with anxiolytic and/or antidepressant potential based on local reports; (II) prepare standard crude extracts; (III) perform phytochemical studies that include sequential partitioning of crude extracts, purification and isolation of phytoconstituents, chemical elucidation or characterization of the isolates, structural modifications or syntheses of new compounds based on chemical structure of their isolates; and (IV) conduct pharmacological analyses of the anti-anxiety and antidepressant properties of the standard crude extracts, fractions, isolated compounds, or derivatives using ex vivo, in vitro, and in vivo assays (e.g., preliminary pharmacological screening, classic animal models of anxiety like the light dark box (LDB) or elevated plus-maze (EPM) tests, etc., or the forced swim test (FST) and tail suspension tests (TST), among others).* These tools have allowed researchers to analyze the possible metabolites responsible for the anxiolytic or antidepressant properties of plants used by different populations, and identify how their mechanisms of action affect the functioning of the central nervous system (CNS). Their studies contribute to advancing scientific understanding of the neurobiology of depression and anxiety, and to developing new pharmacological treatments that may favorably impact public health.

Plants used in traditional medicine contain compounds in their secondary metabolism [13] such as alkaloids, phenols, sterols, carbohydrates, tannins, terpenes, and phytoalexins, all of which have important biological activities [14]. The most widely studied metabolites are terpenes, flavonoids, alkaloids, and sterols, whose mechanisms of action stimulate the serotonergic, noradrenergic, dopaminergic, or GABAergic neurotransmission systems, acting on receptors or the synthetic pathways of neurotransmitters and their transporters. However, they may also stimulate other neurotransmission systems. For example, terpenes can stimulate at the same time serotonergic, dopaminergic, and noradrenergic neurotransmission systems [12] that can produce a similar effect on mood regulation, perhaps leading to an overstimulation that may generate undesirable collateral effects.

This chapter reviews and discusses the findings from research on several metabolites of medicinal plants that have shown potential anxiolytic and antidepressant activities once screened for their biological mechanisms at various levels: receptor, transporter, synthesis, gene, protein, or metabolic. The studies analyzed were identified by a preliminary search in PubMed, Scopus and Ovid for articles on (i) the dose effects and possible mechanisms of action of metabolite(s) isolated from parts of plants with previously identified anxiolytic or antidepressant effects; and (ii) standard chemical tests performed with specific metabolites.

2. Terpenes with antidepressant effects

Terpenes are formed by the union of isoprene units (5 C atoms). Their classification depends on the number of units they contain: 10 C terpenes (two units) are called monoterpenes, while 15 C terpenes (three units) are called sesquiterpenes, and those with 20 C are diterpenes. Triterpenes have 30 C, tetraterpenes have 40 C, and polyterpenes are those with over 8 isoprene units. Studies have evaluated the effect of terpenes isolated from plants, including rosmanol from *Rosmarinus officinalis*, ursolic acid, and oleanolic acid; carnosol from *Artemisa indica*; and linalool and β-pinene from *Litsea glaucescens*. All these terpenes have proven antidepressant effects. Abdelhalim et al. [15] isolated rosmanol, an ethyl acetate diterpene, from *R. officinalis*. A single acute dose of 30 or 100 mg/kg i.p. of rosmanol in male Swiss mice produced an antidepressant effect on the FST and TST. The 100-mg/kg dose produced an effect similar to that of a 60-mg/kg dose of imipramine on the FST. Their study also tested the acute toxicity of administering 50, 150, and 200 mg/kg, i.p., of rosmanol. Some signs of toxic effects on grooming behavior were observed, as well as hyperactivity, sedation, respiratory arrest, convulsions, and locomotor activity. However, no cases of lethality or variations in the amount of food and water ingested were reported.

Other terpenes with antidepressant properties include phenolic diterpene, carnosol, and pentacyclic triterpenoids like betulinic, oleanolic, and ursolic acids.

Metabolite	Extract from plant/part of plant (common name)	Posology (administration way, doses, and duration of treatment)	Experimental subject	Experimental model	Identified effect	Mechanisms of action	References
Alkaloids							
Harmine 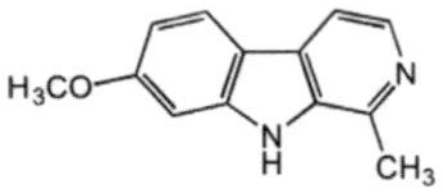	Harmine	i.p. 15 mg/kg/day for 7 days i.p. 5, 10, and 15 mg/kg/day for 7 days	Stressed rats CUMS (60 days old) No stressed rats (60 days old)	• Sucrose preference test • Forced swim test	Antidepressant-like effect in the CUMS model Antidepressant effect with both doses	NE NE	[62]
Mitragynine 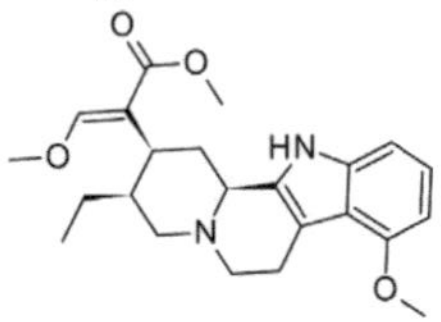	Separated and purified from *Mitragyna speciosa*	i.p 5, 10, and 30 mg/kg a single dose	Male mice	• Tail suspension test • Forced swim test	Antidepressant effect with 10 and 30 mg/kg	Modulating neuroendocrine axis HPA	[67]
Evodiamine 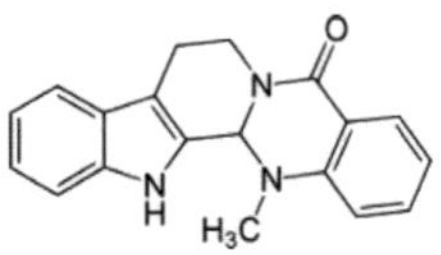	Evodiamine (*Evodia fructus*, *Evodia rutaecarpa* Benth., Rutaceae)	v.o 10–20 mg/kg for 14 days	Male Sprague–Dawley rats (180–220 g)	• Sucrose preference test • Forced swim test	Antidepressant-like effect in the CUMS model	NE	[69]
Protopine	Protopine hydrochloride was synthesized from Protopine *Dactylicapnos scandens*	Doses of 3.75 mg/kg, 7.5 mg/kg and 30 mg/kg	Male BALB/cj mice (20–24 g)	• Tail suspension test	Antidepressant effects with 30 mg/kg	Inhibitor of serotonin transporter and noradrenaline transporter	[71]

Metabolite	Extract from plant/part of plant (common name)	Posology (administration way, doses, and duration of treatment)	Experimental subject	Experimental model	Identified effect	Mechanisms of action	References
Terpenes							
Rosmanol 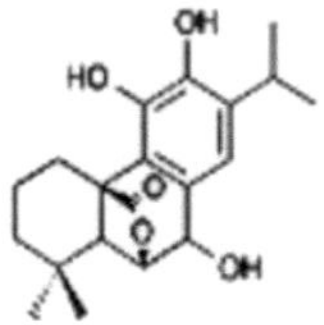	Ethyl acetate extract of *Rosmarinus officinalis* (Rosemary)	i.p. 30 and 100 mg/kg a single dose	Male Swiss mice (20–30 g)	• Forced swim test • Tail suspension test	Antidepressant effect with both doses 100 mg/kg like with imipramine Antidepressant effect with both doses	NE	[15]
Linalool 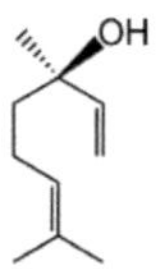 (−)-Linalool 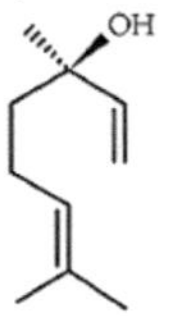	Found shrub such as *Litsea glaucescens* in these studies used chemical standard	i.p. 100 mg/kg a single dose i.p. (10, 50, 100, and 200 mg/kg, a single dose)	Male ICR mice (27–33 g) Male Swiss mice (30–40 g)	• Forced swim test • Tail suspension test	Antidepressant effect with 100 mg/kg Antidepressant effect with 100 and 200 mg/kg	Serotonergic mechanism by 5-HT1A receptors Noradrenergic mechanism by α2-adrenoceptor NE	[22] [21]
(1S)-(−)-β-pinene 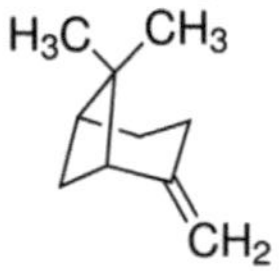	Found shrub such as *Litsea glaucescens*	i.p. 100 mg/kg a single dose	Male ICR mice (27–33 g)	• Forced swim test	Antidepressant effect with 100 mg/kg	Serotonergic mechanism by 5-HT_{1A} receptors Noradrenergic mechanism by activation of the β-adrenoceptor and regulate noradrenergic neurotransmission Dopaminergic mechanisms by activation of D1 receptors	[22]

Metabolite	Extract from plant/part of plant (common name)	Posology (administration way, doses, and duration of treatment)	Experimental subject	Experimental model	Identified effect	Mechanisms of action	References
Ursolic acid 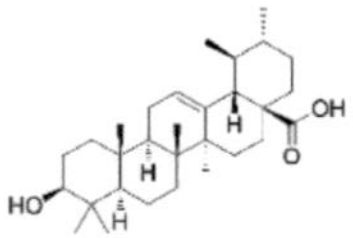 Oleanolic acid 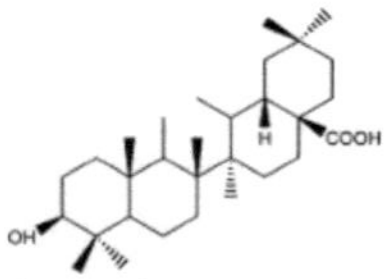 Carnosol 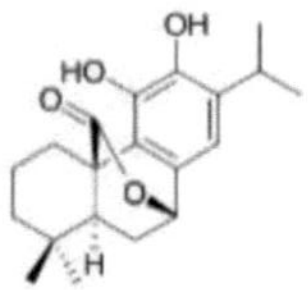	Methanol extract of *Artemisa indica* in the chloroform fraction (Mugwort)	i.p. 10, 30, and 100 mg/kg in a single dose for metabolite independently	Male Swiss mice (20–30 g)	• Forced swim test • Tail suspension test	Antidepressant effect with all doses of three metabolites without effect in locomotor activity 100 mg/kg of ursolic acid was similar to imipramine (60 mg/kg) Antidepressant effect with all doses of three metabolites	Suggest a GABAergic mechanisms in α1β2γ2L $GABA_A$ receptors	[17]
Carnosol 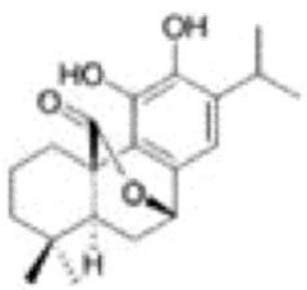 Betulinic acid 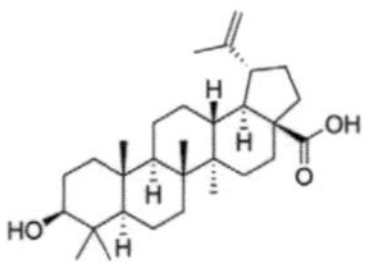	Crude extract of stems and leaves of *Rosmarinus officinalis* and identified and isolation of the hexane fraction (carnosol) and of the ethyl acetate fraction (betulinic acid)	p.o. 0.01, 0.1, 1, and 10 mg/kg, in a single dose p.o. 0.1, 1, and 10 mg/kg, in a single dose	Male Swiss mice (45–50 g, 60–70 days old)	• Tail suspension test	Carnosol produced an antidepressant effect with 0.01 and 0.1 mg/kg, while betulinic acid only with 10 mg/kg	NE	[16]

Metabolite	Extract from plant/part of plant (common name)	Posology (administration way, doses, and duration of treatment)	Experimental subject	Experimental model	Identified effect	Mechanisms of action	References
Ursolic acid 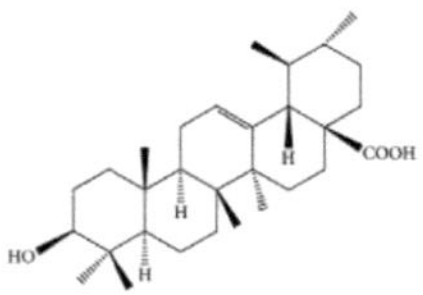	Crude extract of stems and leaves of *Rosmarinus officinalis* and identified in ethyl acetate fraction	p.o. 0.1, 1, and 10 mg/kg, in a single dose p.o. 0.001, 0.01, 0.1, 1, and 10 mg/kg, in a single dose	Male Swiss mice (20–30 g, 60–70 days old)	• Forced swim test • Tail suspension test	Antidepressant effect with 10 mg/kg similar to bupropion (10 mg/kg) Antidepressant effect with 0.01 and 0.1 mg/kg were similar to fluoxetine (10 mg/kg), imipramine (1 mg/kg), and bupropion (10 mg/kg)	NE Suggest a probable dopaminergic mechanism by D1 and D2 receptor	[18]
Ursolic acid 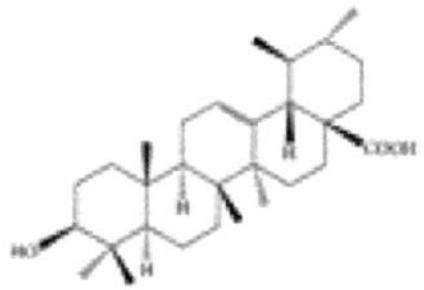	Chemical standard	0.001 and 0.1 mg/kg	Swiss mice (35–45 g, 55–60 days old) of either sex homogeneously distributed	• Tail suspension test	Antidepressant effects with 0.1 mg/kg alone and in combination with pretreatment with PCPA 100 mg/kg, i.p., 4 days 0.001 mg/kg of ursolic acid and 5 mg/kg of fluoxetine produced a pharmacological synergism	Suggest mechanism serotonergic by synthesis of 5-HT and activation of 5-HT_{1A}	[19]
Terpinene-4-ol γ-terpinene Transsabinenehydrate α-terpinene α-terpinolene Cis-sabinenehydrate β-phellandrene ρ-cymene trans-caryophyllene (E)-p-menth-2-en-1-ol bicyclogermacrene β-myrcene	*Origanum majorana* essential oil (OMEO)	The OMEO was made up of 24 compounds Terpinene-4-ol (32.69%) γ-terpinene (12.88%) Transsabinenehydrate (8.47%) α-terpinene (7.98%) sabinene (6.21%) α-terpineol (5.25%) α-terpinolene (3.36%) Cis-sabinenehydrate (2.92%) β-phellandrene (2.64%) ρ-cymene (2.32%) trans-caryophyllene (2.31%) (E)-p-menth-2-en-1-ol	Male mice (20–30 g)	• Forced swim test	Antidepressant effect with 40 and 80 mg/kg of OMEO 80 mg/kg de OMEO was more effective	Dopaminergic mechanisms by activation of D1 and D2 receptors Serotonergic mechanisms by activation of 5-HT_{1A} and 5-HT_{2A} receptors, increases 5-HT synthesis Noradrenergic mechanism by activation of α1 and α2-adrenoceptors They regulate brain monoamine neurotransmitters	[20]

Metabolite	Extract from plant/part of plant (common name)	Posology (administration way, doses, and duration of treatment)	Experimental subject	Experimental model	Identified effect	Mechanisms of action	References
		(2.25%) Bicyclogermacrene (1.60%) β-myrcene (1.49%) These anointed for 92.37% of the yield, while the other detected components represented <1.0% in each case. 10, 20, 40, and 80 mg/kg of OMEO in a single dose					
Hesperidin 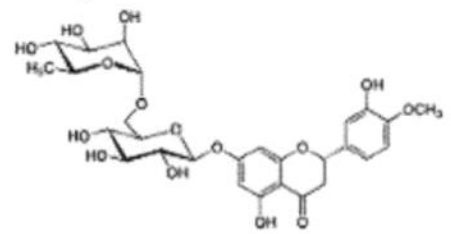	Commercial flavonoid (Sigma Chemical)	i.p 0.01, 0.1, 0.3, and 1 mg/kg, for 21 days	Male Swiss mice	• Tail suspension test	Antidepressant effect with all doses evaluated	Increase in BDNF concentrations in the hippocampus	[42]
Quercetin 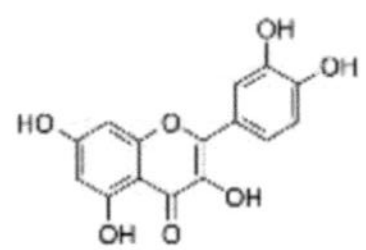	Commercial flavonoid (Sigma Chemical)	25 mg/kg, for 14 days	Bulbectomized mice	• Tail suspension test • Forced swim test	Antidepressant effect with 25 mg/kg	Lipid hydroperoxide content (LOOH) levels were reversed by quercetin; antidepressant-like effects seem to occur by modulation of glutamate and nitric oxide	[37]
Kaempferitrin 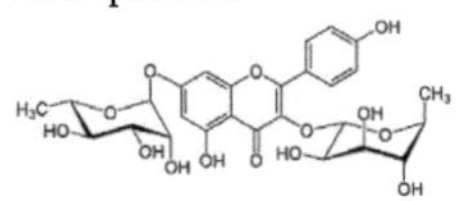	Isolation of aerial parts of *Justicia spicigera*	1.0, 5.0, 10, and 20 mg/kg doses	Male Swiss Webster mice	• Tail suspension test • Forced swim test	Antidepressant effect with 5.0, 10, and 20 mg/kg doses	The activation of 5HT1A receptors and the synthesis of 5-HT are mandatory to produce effect of noradrenergic mechanism by α2- adrenoceptor agonism	[95]

Metabolite	Extract from plant/part of plant (common name)	Posology (administration way, doses, and duration of treatment)	Experimental subject	Experimental model	Identified effect	Mechanisms of action	References
Quercetin 4'-O-glucoside 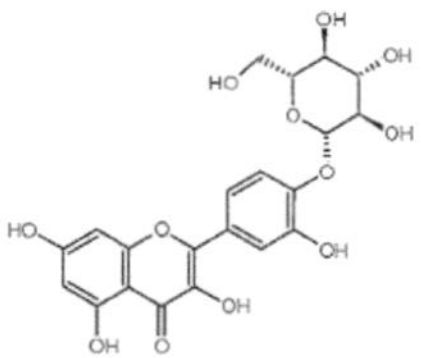	Bulbs of *Allium cepa* var	p.o. 50 and 100 mg/kg extract. Once daily for 7 days	Swiss albino mice of either sex	• Forced swim test	Antidepressant effect with 50 and 100 mg/kg	Effect might be attributed to its anti-oxidant properties, MAO-A inhibition, and consequent increase in brain 5-HT levels	[36]
Genistein 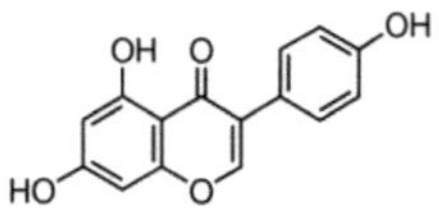	Commercial Genistein (Ze Lang Biotechnology)	p.o. 5–45 mg/kg, (once per day for 3 weeks)	Male ICR mice	• Forced swim test • Tail suspension test	Antidepressant effect with 15 and 45 mg/kg 45 mg/kg is similar to imipramine 15 mg/kg	Genistein was potentiated by co-treatment with 8-OH-DPAT ($5\text{-}HT_{1A}$ receptor agonist)	[33]
Baicalin 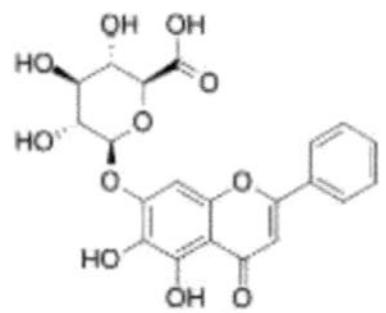	Commercial flavonoid (Nanjing, China)	60 mg/kg	Male ICR mice	• Sucrose preference test	Antidepressant effect	Through a mechanism to promote the differentiation of neurons, and the transformation into mature neurons and their survival via the Akt/FOXG1 pathway	[43]
Naringin 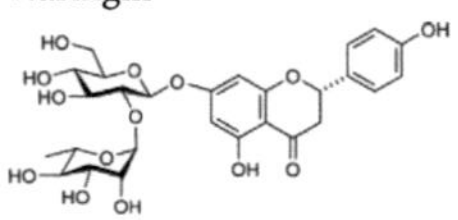	Commercial Naringin (Sigma-Aldrich)	i.p. 2.5, 5, and 10 mg/kg, once daily for 7 days	Male Swiss mice	• Forced swim test	Antidepressant effects	Maybe by increased neuro-antioxidant and cholinergic activities and it significantly decreased malondialdehyde and nitrite concentrations, suggesting the involvement of oxidative/nitrosative pathways	[44]

Metabolite	Extract from plant/part of plant (common name)	Posology (administration way, doses, and duration of treatment)	Experimental subject	Experimental model	Identified effect	Mechanisms of action	References
Fisetin 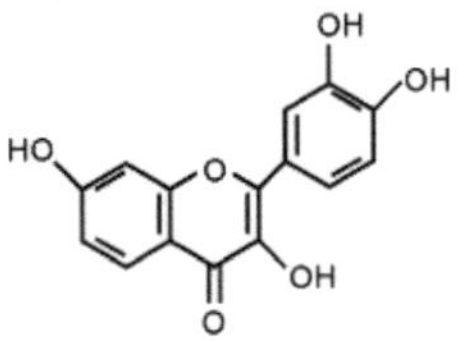	Commercial Fisetin (Sigma-Aldrich)	p.o. 5 mg/kg, with 1–2 weeks of treatment	Male adult ICR mice	• Tail suspension test • Forced swim test	Antidepressant effect	Maybe by activation of TrkB signaling in the hippocampus suggesting pro-neurogenesis effects of fisetin in the hippocampus	[40]
Sterols							
Fucosterol 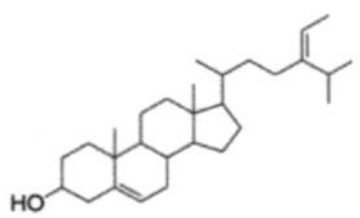	Ethanol extract of *Sargassum fusiforme* (algas)	i.p. 10, 20, 30, and 40 mg/kg	Male Balb/e mice (20 ± 2 g)	• Forced swim test • Tail suspension test	Antidepressant effect with dose 20 and 30 mg/kg like fluoxetine	Increase in CNS 5HT, NA, and BDNF levels	[92]
β-Sitosterol 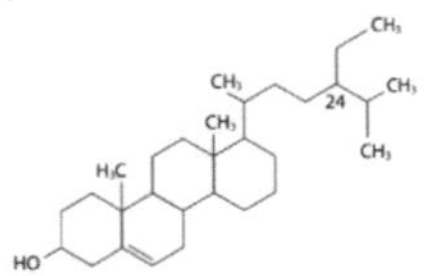	Ethanol extract of *Sargassum horneri*	i.p. 10, 20, and 30 mg/kg, for 7 days	Male Kun Ming mice (20 ± 2 g)	• Forced swim test • Tail suspension test	Antidepressant effect with dose 20 mg/kg β-sitosterol and 200 mg/kg sterols total like fluoxetine	Increase in CNS 5-HT, NA β-sitosterol increases 5-HIAA levels	[93]
α-Spinasterol 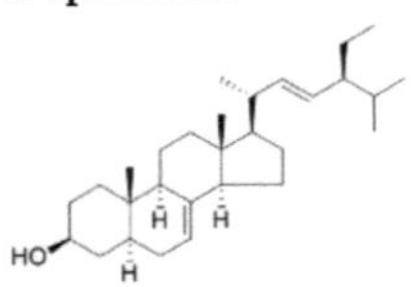	Toronto Research Chemicals Inc., Canada	i.p. 1 and 2 mg/kg	Male albino Swiss mice (23–25 g)	• Forced swim test	Antidepressant effect with dose 1 and 2 mg/kg	TRPV1 antagonistic effects	[90]

Metabolite	Extract from plant/part of plant (common name)	Posology (administration way, doses, and duration of treatment)	Experimental subject	Experimental model	Identified effect	Mechanisms of action	References
β-Amirine 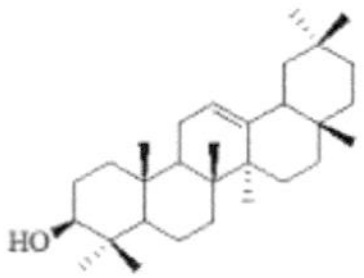 α-Amirine 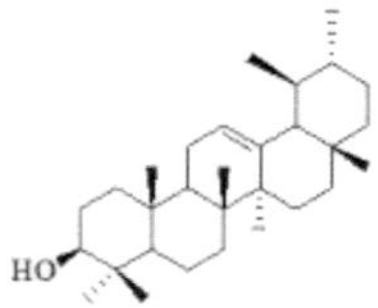	Hexane–ethyl acetate extracts from *Protium heptaphyllum*	p.o. 1, 2.5, and 5 mg/kg	Male Swiss mice (20–30 g)	• Forced swim test	Antidepressant effect with dose 2.5 and 5 mg/kg	NE	[94]

NE = no explorated.

Table 1.
Secondary metabolites with antidepressant properties in preclinical study.

Metabolite	Extract from plant/part of plant (common name)	Posology (administration way, doses and duration of treatment)	Experimental subject	Experimental model	Identified effect	Mechanisms of action	References
Alkaloids							
Gelsemine 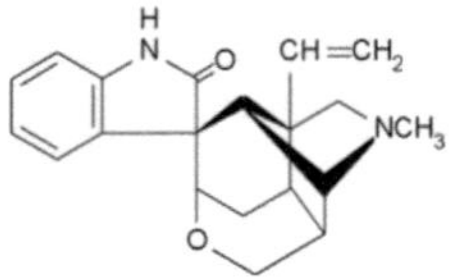 Koumine 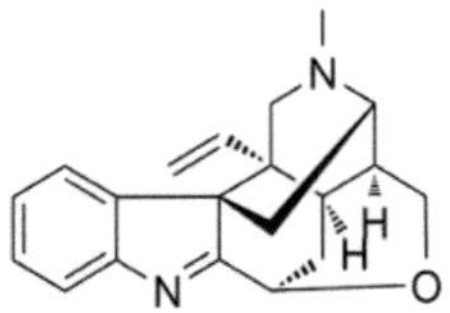 Gelsevirine 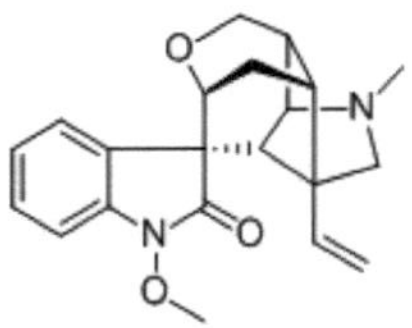	Isolated from *Gelsemium elegans* Benth	s.c. gelsemine, koumine and gelsevirine 0.4, 2, and 10 mg/kg s.c. gelsenicine 0.8, 4, or 20 μg/kg	Male mice (24–26 g)	• Elevated plus maze • Light/dark box	Anxiolytic activity with all doses	Mechanism may be involved in the glycine receptor	[72]
Gelsemine 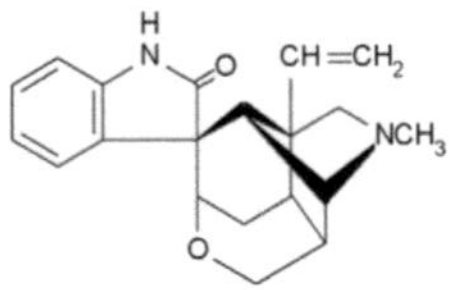	Hydroalcoholic solution of *Gelsemium elegans* Benth	i.p. 500 μl ($10–^{6}$, $10–^{10}$, or $10–^{14}$ M) for 7 days	Male Sprague–Dawley rats (250–300 g)	• Elevated plus maze	Anxiolytic activity with $10–^{6}$ and $10–^{10}$ M	NE	[73]

Metabolite	Extract from plant/part of plant (common name)	Posology (administration way, doses and duration of treatment)	Experimental subject	Experimental model	Identified effect	Mechanisms of action	References
Koumine 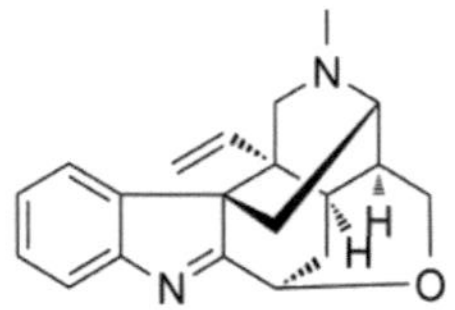	Separated and purified from *Gelsemium elegans*	s.c. 0.167, 0.5, or 1.5 mg/kg Only one administration	Male Wistar rats (6–8 weeks and 180–220 g)	• Vogel conflict test	Anxiolytic effect with all doses	NE	[74]
Berberine (isoquinoline alkaloid) 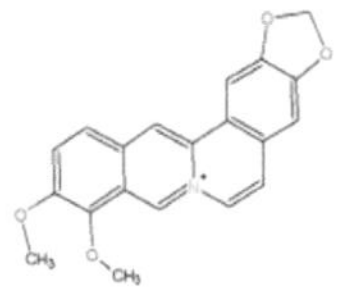	Berberine hydrochloride	v.o. 100 mg/kg/day for 21 days	Male Wistar rats (200–250 g)	• Elevated plus maze	Anxiety-like behaviors in addiction	Modulation of neuropeptide oxytocin and its receptor	[59]
Terpenes							
Rosmanol 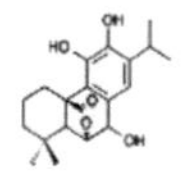	Ethyl acetate extract of *Rosmarinus officinalis* (Rosemary)	i.p. 1, 10, 30, and 100 mg/kg Only one administration	Male Swiss mice (20–30 g)	• Elevated plus maze • Light/dark box	Anxiolytic effect with 10, 30, and 100 mg/kg 10 and 30 mg/kg like diazepam (1 mg/kg)	Suggest a GABAergic mechanisms in $GABA_A$ receptors PTZ (20 mg/kg), but not Flumazenil (2.5 mg/kg) blocked the anxiolytic effect of 10 mg/kg of rosmanol in the elevated plus maze	[15]
Linalool oxide 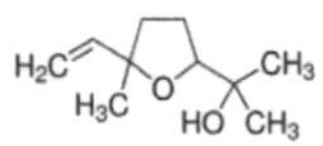	Frequently found aromatic plants such as *Lavandula angustifolia* Mill., *Melissa officinalis* L., Rosmarinus officinalis L., and *Cymbopogon citratus* DC	Inhalation of linalool oxide emulsion 0.65%, 1.25%, 2.5%, and 5.0% w/w. 7 min of exposure to the inhalation chamber	Male Swiss mice (20–30 g)	• Elevated plus maze • Light/dark box • Rota-rod test	Anxiolytic effect with all doses without effect in coordination motriz	NE	[28]

Metabolite	Extract from plant/part of plant (common name)	Posology (administration way, doses and duration of treatment)	Experimental subject	Experimental model	Identified effect	Mechanisms of action	References
Ursolic acid 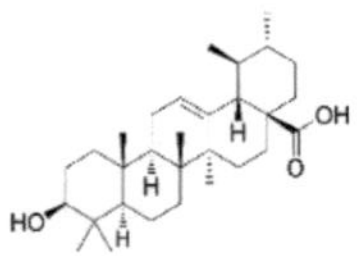 Oleanolic acid 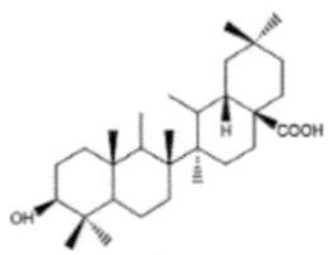 Carnosol 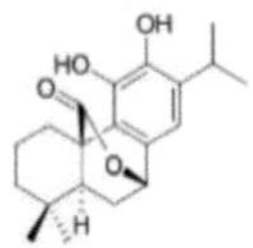	Methanol extract of whole *Artemisa indica* in the chloroform fraction (Mugwort)	i.p. 1, 10, 30, and 100 mg/kg Only one administration	Male Swiss mice (20–30 g)	• Elevated plus maze • Light/dark box	Anxiolytic effect with 10, 30, and 100 mg/kg of the three metabolites without effect in locomotor activity 30 and 100 mg/kg of the three metabolites are like diazepam (1 mg/kg)	Flumazenil (2.5 mg/kg) blocked the anxiolytic effect of 10 mg/kg of the three metabolites in elevated plus maze test Suggest a GABAergic mechanisms in α1β2γ2L $GABA_A$ receptors	[17]
Songorine 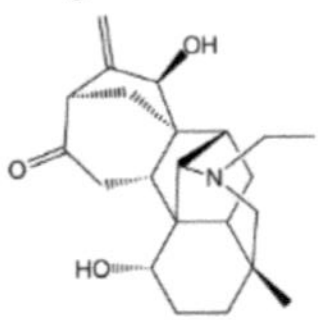	The chloroform extract obtained from the aerial part of wolfsbane (*A. barbatum* Pers.)	p.o. 2.5 and 0.25 mg/kg, for 5 days	Male CBA/CaLac mice (20–22 g)	• Vogel conflict test	Anxiolytic activity with 0.25 mg/kg produced exceeding that of phenazepam Without sedative effect	NE	[29]
p-Cymene + thymol	Ethyl acetate extract of *Lippia graveolens* leaves	i.p. 3 mg/kg	Male CD-1 mice (25–30 g)	• Hole-board test • Elevated plus maze	Anxiolytic effect	NE	[24]

Metabolite	Extract from plant/part of plant (common name)	Posology (administration way, doses and duration of treatment)	Experimental subject	Experimental model	Identified effect	Mechanisms of action	References
Flavonoids							
Quercetin 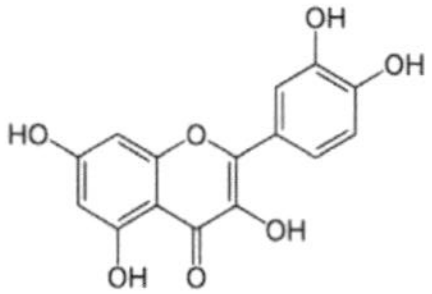 Rutin 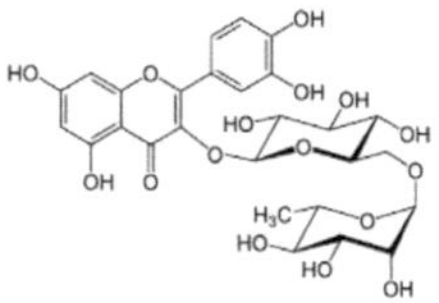 Isoquercitrin 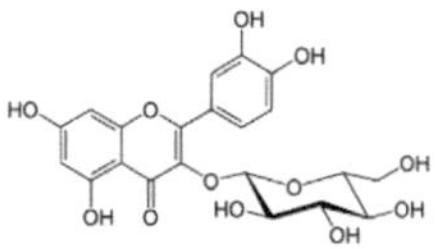	Flowers and bracts of *Tilia americana* L.	All i.p. mixes of quercetin (20 mg/kg), isoquercitrin (2 mg/kg), and rutin (15.70 mg/kg)	Male CD-1 mice	• Hole-board test • Elevated plus maze	Anxiolytic-like effects producing a significant diminution in head dips during the hole-board test, an increase in time spent at the open-side arms in the plus-maze	The involvement of GABAergic and serotonergic receptors. Flumazenil and WAY100635, inhibited the anxiolytic-like effects of the flavonoid mixture in the plus-maze test, while WAY100635 showed a significant decrease in the number of explorations in the hole-board test	[46]
Formononetin 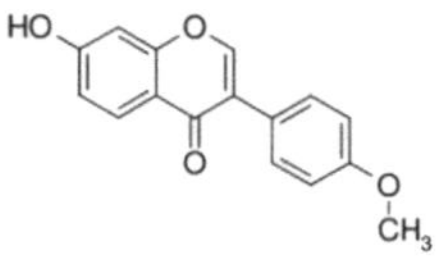	Formononetin from *Trifolium pratense L.*	25 mg/kg for 8 consecutive days	C57BL/6 male mice	• Elevated plus maze	Formononetin relieved CFA-induced anxiety-like behaviors in mice	A mechanism based on the inhibition of hyperexcitability and inflammation in the basolateral amygdala is suggested through the inhibition of NMDA receptor and CREB-binding protein (CBP)	[47]

Metabolite	Extract from plant/part of plant (common name)	Posology (administration way, doses and duration of treatment)	Experimental subject	Experimental model	Identified effect	Mechanisms of action	References
Theaflavins	TF40, a crude theaflavin extract	p.o 1 or 5 mg/kg theaflavins, once a day for 5 days for EPM and once a day for 6 days for LDB	DDY male mice	• Elevated plus maze • Light/dark box	5 mg/kg theaflavins show anxiolytic-like effects in both models. In EPM, the time spent in the open arms was significantly increased, while the time spent and the number of entries in the light box increased	Theaflavin increased the levels of 3,4-dihydroxyphenylacetic acid (DOPAC) and the ratios of DOPAC/DA and (DOPAC + homovanillic acids)/DA indicating DA turnover, in the frontal cortex	[48]
Chrysin 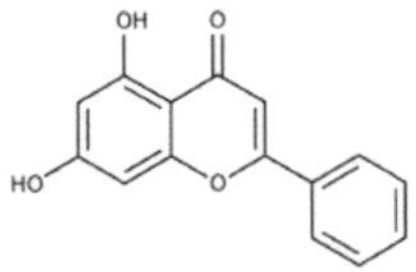	Commercial Chrysin (Sigma-Aldrich)	(0.5, 1, 2, and 4 mg/kg)	Adult female Wistar rats in a model of surgical menopause	• Light/dark box • Elevated plus maze	2 and 4 mg/kg produced anxiolytic-like effects. Increased the total time spent in the light compartment in rats with the long-term absence of ovarian hormones. With respect to the elevated plus maze, chrysin (2 mg/kg) increased the time spent on the open arms	$GABA_A$ receptor activation partial, pretreatment with picrotoxin (1 mg/kg), did not block the anxiolytic-like effects of chrysin	[49]
Puerarin 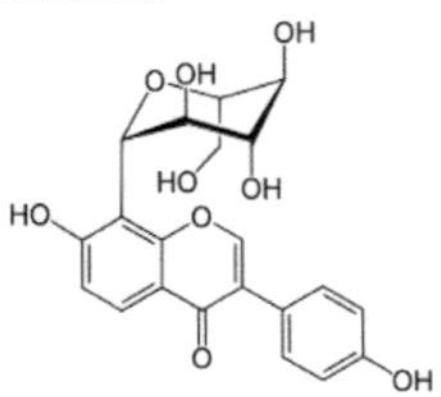	Commercial Puerarin (Sigma-Aldrich)	p.o. 30, 60, and 120 mg/kg	Male Sprague–Dawley rats	• Elevated plus maze • Vogel conflict test	Anxiolytic-like effects were produced by puerarin (60 and 120 mg/kg, i.g)	It's suggested that puerarin (60 and 120 mg/kg, i.g.) produced an increase of allopregnanolone and serotonin (5-HT) in the prefrontal cortex	[50]

Metabolite	Extract from plant/part of plant (common name)	Posology (administration way, doses and duration of treatment)	Experimental subject	Experimental model	Identified effect	Mechanisms of action	References
Genistein 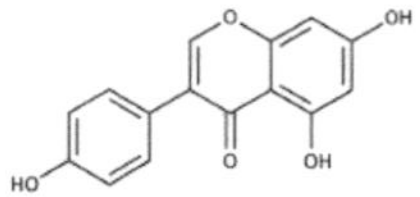	Commercial Genistein (Sigma-Aldrich)	i.p. 2–8 mg/kg, for 7 days	Sprague–Dawley male rats	• Elevated plus maze	Anxiolytic-like effects were produced by genistein (2–8 mg/kg)	Significantly increased total time spent in open arms in a dose-dependent manner	[53]
6-Methoxyflavanone 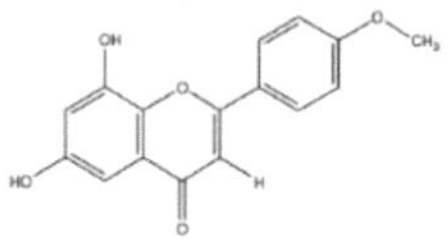	Commercial 6-methoxyflavanone (Sigma-Aldrich)	i.p. 10, 30, 50, and 100 mg/kg	BALB/c mice of both sex	• Elevated plus maze • Staircase test	6-methoxyflavanone (10, 30, and 50 mg/kg) spent appreciably longer in the open and arms and on the central platform like diazepam. In staircase test, both diazepam and flavonoid 6-MeOF (10 and 30 mg/kg) reduced the incidence of rearing without decreasing the number of steps ascended	α1-subunit containing $GABA_A$ receptor mediated sedative action of the 6-methoxyflavanone	[56]
Rutin 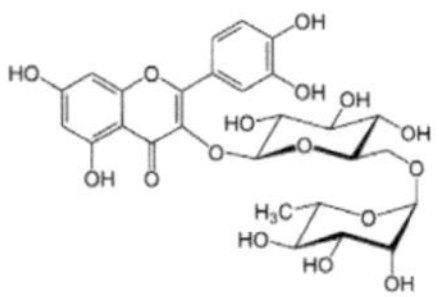	Commercial Rutin (Sigma-Aldrich)	(i.p.) 30, 100, 300, 562, and 1000 mg/kg microinjected into the basolateral amygdala (16 nmol/4 μl, intracerebral)	Male Wistar rats	• Elevated plus maze	Anxiolytic-like effects in rutin (300–1000 mg/kg) significantly and dose manner dependently increased (3–6-fold) the number of entries to the open arms and the time spent in this significantly increased in a dose-dependent manner	Anxiolytic-like effects are partly modulated by $GABA_A$ receptors in the basolateral amygdala. Flumazenil partly antagonized the effects of systemic rutin	[57]

Metabolite	Extract from plant/part of plant (common name)	Posology (administration way, doses and duration of treatment)	Experimental subject	Experimental model	Identified effect	Mechanisms of action	References
Viscosine 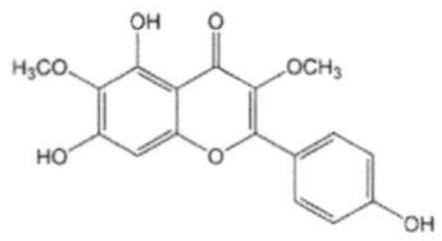	*Dodonaea viscosa* (Linn)	i.p. 10, 30, and 100 mg/kg	Male Swiss mice	• Elevated plus maze • Light/dark box	Viscosin increased the % entries and % time spent in the open arms	Anxiolytic effect of viscosine are likely mediated via its positive allosteric modulatory action of GABA at different $GABA_A$ receptor subtypes	[58]
Sterols							
α-Spinasterol 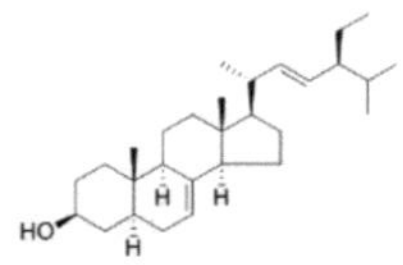	Toronto Research Chemicals Inc., Canada	i.p. 1 and 2 mg/kg	Male albino Swiss mice (23–25 g)	• Elevated plus maze • Light/dark box	No effects were found (0.5, 1, and 2 mg/kg)	NE	[90]
β-Amirine 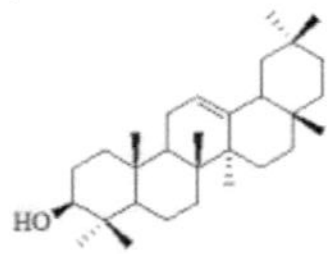 α-Amirine 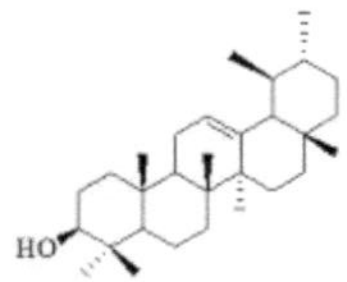	Hexane–ethyl acetate from *Protium heptaphyllum*	p.o. 10, 25, and 50 mg/kg	Male Swiss mice (20–30 g)	• Elevated plus maze	Anxiolytic effect with dose 10–25 mg/kg like diazepam	Mechanisms GABAérgic by $GABA_A$ receptors in the subunit α1	[94]

NE = no explorated.

Table 2.
Secondary metabolites with anxiolytic properties in preclinical study.

Carnosol generated an antidepressant-like effect at doses of 0.01 and 0.1 mg/kg [16] on TST, and 10, 30, and 100 mg/kg, i.p., on TST and FST, as did the oleanolic and ursolic acids. Meanwhile, 100 mg/kg of ursolic acid showed an effect similar to that of imipramine at 60 mg/kg [17]. Betulinic acid at 10 mg/kg was evaluated in male mice on TST [16]. None of those metabolites had effects on locomotor activity. Ursolic acid at doses of 0.01 and 0.1 mg/kg produced an effect similar to that of fluoxetine (10 mg/kg), imipramine (1 mg/kg), and bupropion (10 mg/kg) on TST [18]. Only the 10-mg/kg dose had an antidepressant effect on FST, which was similar to that of bupropion at 10 mg/kg. Studies exploring the mechanism of action of ursolic acid found the involvement of D1 and D2 receptors and a pharmacological synergism with bupropion at 1 mg/kg, p.o. (dual dopamine/noradrenaline reuptake inhibitor, DDNRI) [18], 5 mg/kg of fluoxetine, or 2 mg/kg of reboxetine (SRNI) [19]. They also observed a related increase in noradrenaline and dopamine synthesis on TST [19]. These findings are noteworthy because they suggest the possibility that various mechanisms of action may be stimulated by the same metabolite.

A study of the essential oil of *Origanum majorana* (OMEO) identified 14 component terpenes that represented 92.32% of yield. The five components that were more abundant in OMEO were terpinene-4-ol (32.69%), γ-terpinene (12.88%), trans-sabinene hydrate (8.47%), α-terpinene (7.98%), and sabinene (6.211%). Administered in a single acute dose of 40 or 80 mg/kg, OMEO increased swimming and climbing times in male mice on FST. These findings were interpreted as showing an antidepressant-like effect. In that study [20], pretreatment with antagonist drugs demonstrated that the terpenes act through several mechanisms: first, by activating the dopaminergic receptors D_1 and D_2, the noradrenergic α1- and α2-adrenoceptor, and the $5\text{-}HT_{1A}$ and $5\text{-}HT_{2A}$ receptors, and, second, by activating or increasing 5-HT synthesis and monoamine vesicular storage involved in reducing the immobility time produced by 80 mg/kg of OMEO [20]. A pharmacological synergism at the combined subthreshold OMEO doses of 10 mg/kg plus fluoxetine or imipramine (5 mg/kg, i.p.) was also seen. It reduced immobility time but increased swimming and climbing times, similar effects to those produced by OMEO at 80 mg/kg [20]. (A more detail view about the OMEO components can be reviewed at **Tables 1** and **2** as summary). (R)-(−)-linalool produced antidepressant effects in male mice on TST at a single dose of 100 or 200 mg/kg, i.p., and on FST when administered 3 times at 100 mg/kg, i.p. [21]. That effect was produced by activation of the $5\text{-}HT_{1A}$ receptor and α2-adrenoceptors [22], while (1S)-(−)-β-pinene produced an antidepressant effect after three applications at a dose of 100 mg/kg, i.p., by activating β-adrenoceptors, $5\text{-}HT_{1A}$ and D1-receptors, and noradrenergic neurotransmission in the cerebral cortex [22].

However, due to the terpene's capacity to stimulate several neurotransmission systems—especially high doses of monoterpenes—possible collateral or undesirable effects as serotonergic syndrome need to be explored. The monoterpenic oxide, 1,4-cineole, for example, produced a prodespair effect at doses of 200 mg/kg, i.p., on FST and 400 mg/kg, i.p., and FST and TST, but did not induce any significant deficit in motor coordination on the rota-rod test (RRT). It did, however, have an anxiolytic effect at a dose of 400 mg/kg in male mice evaluated in EPM that was not associated with any sedative effect [23]. These findings require additional study in light of potential depressor effects on the CNS, and to elucidate the mechanisms of action involved.

3. Terpenes with anxiolytic effects: preclinical research

Anxiolytic properties have also been attributed to terpenes. A combination of two monoterpenoids, p-cymene + thymol, both at doses of 3mg/kg i.p., produced anxiolytic effects on the hole-board test (HBT) and EPM [24]. Studies have also demonstrated that (−)-myrtenol, a monoterpenoid alcohol, produced an anxiolytic effect on EPM at doses of 25, 50, and 75 mg/kg, i.p., though only the 25- and 50-mg/kg doses did so on LDB. On both tests, the anxiolytic effect of 25 mg/kg of (−)-myrtenol was mediated by $GABA_A$ receptors [25]. In another study, rosmanol produced an anxiolytic effect at doses of 10, 30, and 100 mg/kg in EPM and LDB, and the 10- and 30-mg/kg doses showed an effect similar to those of diazepam at 1 mg/kg [15]. This mechanism of action acts on $GABA_A$ receptors at a distinct site from the high-affinity benzodiazepine-binding region [15]. Triterpenes as ursolic acid, oleanolic acid, and carnosol produced anxiolytic effects at doses of 10, 30, and 100 mg/kg in EPM and LDB. The effect of the 30- and 100-mg/kg doses of these three metabolites was similar to that of diazepam at 1 mg/kg. No significant effect was seen on locomotor activity. We know that this effect was produced through $GABA_A$ receptors of the $\alpha 1\beta 2\gamma 2L$ conformation because 2.5 mg/kg of flumazenil blocked the anxiolytic effects of 10 mg/kg of all three in EPM [17].

Although most terpenes have a GABAergic mechanism, their action may also occur through the serotonergic system, as evidenced in the study by Costa et al. [26]. In an experiment with male rats, those authors identified that acute administration of 5 mg/kg, p.o., or 14-day repeat doses (1 mg/kg/day), of the essential oil of ripe fruits of *C. aurantium* (Rutaceae) (whose chemical composition includes 98.66% limonene, 0.53% β-myrcene, 0.41% β-pinene, and 0.41% unidentified compounds) produced an anxiolytic-like effect in LDB that was mediated by the serotonergic system through 5-HT1A receptors (WAY 100635 0.5 mg/kg, i.p.), not the GABAergic system (flumazenil 2 mg/kg, i.p.). That study also analyzed the antidepressant effect on FST after oral and inhaled treatment, but found that it did not modify immobility. Their results suggest that distinct mechanisms of action exist for the anxiolytic and antidepressant effects [26]. In this regard, some of the terpenes in certain essential oils produce anxiolytic effects and are often used in aromatherapy to reduce anxiety in animals and humans [27]. Inhaling emulsions of linalool oxide (a monocyclic alcohol) at 0.65, 1.25, 2.5, and 5.0% w/w during 7 min of exposure in the inhalation chamber, for example, produced anxiolytic-like effects in EPM and LDB, but no significant motor deficit on RRT [28].

Finally, songorine, a C20 diterpenoid alkaloid, produced an anxiolytic-like effect at 0.25 mg/kg v.o. for 5 days with greater efficacy than phenazepam on Vogel's conflict test (VCT) [29]. For the terpenes described so far, we know that both the serotonergic and GABAergic systems are involved in their mechanisms of action, and these are the same systems that are activated by other groups of metabolites, such as flavonoids and sterols (see **Tables 1** and **2** for summaries).

4. Flavonoids with antidepressant effects: preclinical research

Flavonoids are the most widely studied active metabolites (for a broad review of research, see German-Ponciano et al. [30]). Genistein is an isoflavone that can cross the blood-brain barrier in mice [31] and rats [32]. Acute oral administration of 5, 15, and 45 mg/kg genistein in male mice did not reduce immobility time on FST or TST, but chronic, dose-dependent administration for 21 days produced antidepressant-like effects on both tests, without affecting locomotor activity [33]. This effect was associated with increased NA and 5-HT concentrations in the hippocampus and frontal cortex, and of 5-HT in the hypothalamus, though it decreased the 5-HTIAA/5-HT ratio in the hippocampus and frontal cortex. These results suggest an inhibition effect of genistein on MAO-A in the hippocampus, frontal cortex, and hypothalamus and on MAO-B in the hippocampus, three brain structures involved in the neurobiology of depression and anxiety. Their results [33] also demonstrate that central depletion of 5-HT reversed the antidepressant effect of genistein, suggesting a critical role of the serotonergic system, specifically through 5-HT_{1A} receptors. It is important to note that these results on the serotonergic metabolic ratio (5-HIAA/5-HT) may be dependent on gonadal hormones. Ovariectomized rats (OVX, surgical removal of both ovaries) showed reduced immobility times on FST after administration of genistein (10 mg/kg, p.o. [34], or by i.m.) [35] for 14 days, but the downward tendency of the serotonergic metabolic ratio caused by FST was only evident in the hippocampus [34]. Sapronov and Kasakova [35] found antidepressant-like effects on FST at the same dose of genistein (10 mg/kg) but in non-ovariectomized rats. That effect was more marked in the metestrus and diestrus phases of the estral cycle, which are characterized by low plasmatic concentrations of ovarian hormones, than during the proestrus and estrus stages with their characteristically high hormone concentrations. This suggests that these hormones play a significant role in the antidepressant effect of genistein.

A similar effect on the serotonergic system and MAO-A activity was found with quercetin 4'-O-glucoside or quercetin administered at doses of 10 and 20 mg/kg, p.o., for 7 days in Swiss albino mice of both sexes. These substances produced antidepressant-like effects in mice on FST as well as those subjected to unpredictable, chronic mild stress (CUMS, a mouse model designed to induce depression) and subsequently evaluated on FST. In that study, a 20-mg/kg dose of quercetin 4'-O-glucoside showed a similar effect to that of fluoxetine at 20 mg/kg, p.o., on FST, with or without prior exposure to CUMS [36]. A consequence of CUMS on the sucrose preference test (SPT, a test used to study anhedonia rodents, the main symptom of depression in humans) is a decrease in the consumption of a sweetened solution. In these sense, both doses of quercetin 4'-O-glucoside reverted this effect, and interpreted as being antidepressant. Other consequences of CUMS are metabolic, for example, excessive production of reactive oxygen species that was evidenced by higher brain thiobarbituric acid reactive species (TBARS). Compromising endogenous anti-oxidants, like reduced glutathione (GSH), enhances MAO-A activity in the brain and, consequently, depletes monoamine levels there, especially serotonin 5-HT. The effects observed in that study were blocked by 21 days of treatment with 10 and 20 mg/kg of quercetin 4'-O-glucoside [36], suggesting a possible mechanism of action with an antioxidant effect that impedes ROS production. Another study [37] found that 10 mg/kg of quercetin administered for 14 days reduced immobility time on TST, but not FST, while doses of 25 and 50 mg/kg produced this effect in female mice on both tests. The mechanisms of action were explored on TST, where i.c.v. administration of N-methyl-D-aspartate (NMDA at 0.1 pmol/site) and L-arginine (at 750 mg/kg, i.p., a nitric oxide inhibitor) blocked the antidepressant effect of quercetin. Hence, the antidepressant-like effect of quercetin may involve inhibiting NMDA receptors to decrease intracellular calcium that, in turn, inhibits the protein calmodulin, which then inhibits neuronal nitric oxide synthase to decrease nitric oxide levels (NO). This hypothesis is supported by the finding that administering methylene blue (a NO synthase inhibitor) at 20 mg/kg, i.p., and soluble guanylate cyclase or 7-nitroindazole (another NO synthase inhibitor) at 50 mg/kg, i.p., improved quercetin's antidepressant-like effect on TST. This indicates that the antidepressant effect may be dependent on limiting NO synthesis, either by inhibiting the enzyme or by reducing NO production, perhaps via decreased cyclic guanosine monophosphate (cGMP), since sildenafil (a phosphodiesterase 5 selective inhibitor that increases cGMP levels) also canceled this effect [37].

A model of depression induced by olfactory bulbectomy (OB, surgical removal of the olfactory bulbs) reduced the latency to immobility and increased immobility time on FST and TST. This was accompanied by an increase in the levels of the markers of oxidative stress, for example, 116% in the case of lipid hydroperoxide content (LOOH) in the hippocampus. This effect was reverted by 52.25% by administering 25 mg/kg of genistein in the content of LOOH, as observed on the immobility on FST and TST. In sham rats only (*i.e.*, animals subjected to the same surgical procedure but without resection of the olfactory bulbs), genistein reduced glutathione (GSH) levels, in that study by 65.94%. The authors [37] explained that "the reduction of GSH levels caused by OB and, surprisingly, quercetin, can be explained by the fact that glutathione peroxidase, in addition to reducing H_2O_2, decreases lipid and nonlipid hydroperoxides at the expense of GSH, causing it to become oxidized and giving rise to glutathione disulfide. Therefore, it is suggested that LOOH activated glutathione peroxidase which, in turn, oxidized GSH to normalize LOOH levels". In this area, increased levels of the markers of oxidative stress in major depression have been associated with poor response to antidepressant treatment [38]. Therefore, a therapy that reduces the levels of markers of oxidative stress and produces antidepressant effects could be a promising form of treatment.

Additional mechanisms of the antidepressant action of flavonoids have been explored. Administering chrysin for 14 days at a dose of 20 mg/kg, for example, increased grooming time in male OB C57B/6J mice evaluated on the splash test (ST), where 200 ml of a 10% sucrose solution is squirted on the mouse's snout to initiate grooming behavior. Here, greater grooming time is considered an antidepressant effect. Doses of 5 and 20 mg/kg impeded an increase in immobility time by these OB mice on FST, but increased 5-HT and brain-derived neurotrophic factor concentrations in the hippocampus [39]. In another study, fisetin administered at 5 mg/kg v.o. increased activation of the tropomyosin kinase B receptor (TrkB) by signaling and increasing its phosphorylation in the hippocampus. This suggests that fisetin produced pro-neurogenesis [40] related to its antidepressant effect on FST and TST after 1 or 2 weeks of treatment with a relatively short therapeutic latency compared to clinically-effective antidepressants. Fisetin also reversed depression-like behaviors induced by spatial restraint stress in mice evaluated on FST and TST [40]. Other studies have found that the chemical standard dihydromyricetin activated the ERK1/2-CREB pathway and increased glycogen synthase kinase-3 beta (GSK-3β) phosphorylation at ser-9 with upregulation of BDNF expression in the hippocampus, while inhibiting neuroinflammation. These findings may be related to the antidepressant effect seen on TST and FST after once-daily administration of 10 and 20 mg/kg, v.o. for 3 days, but not after a single acute dose [41]. Interestingly, dihydromyricetin reverted the depressogenic effect caused by CUMS in mice subjected to SPT and FST, or TST, only after administration of once daily for 7 days, but not 3 days [41]. Another flavonoid analyzed is hesperidin, which increased BDNF levels in the hippocampus after administration of once daily for 21 days (0.3 and 1 mg/kg, i.p.). These doses produced an antidepressant effect on TST similar to fluoxetine (32 mg/kg i.p.) and imipramine (15 mg/kg, i.p.). Another research has also verified that when applied acutely (1 mg/kg after 30 min) or chronically (0.1, 0.3, and 1 mg/kg for 21 days) hesperidin significantly decreased nitrate/nitrite (NOX) levels in the hippocampus of mice, suggesting a possible inhibition of the L-arginine-NO-cGMP pathway [42].

Another flavonoid that has shown effects on the CNS is baicalin, which may promote neuronal differentiation through neuronal maduration and ensure their survival via the associated Akt/FOXG1 pathway, which stimulates dendrite elongation. This is related to findings that indicated that, after 6 weeks of treatment, a 60-mg/kg dose of baicalin had an effect similar to that of fluoxetine (15 mg/kg, v.o.), because it reverted the decrease of sucrose intake on SPT and the increase in immobility on TST produced by CUMS [43]. Another flavonoid that associates antidepressant and antioxidant effects is naringin, which reduced immobility on FST at doses of 2.5, 5, and 10 mg/kg given for 7 days. The antidepressant effect of these doses correlated with enhanced cholinergic transmission due to a decrease in the activity of the enzyme acetylcholinesterase and of the antioxidant defense systems caused by higher GSH levels, as well as an increase in the activity of superoxide dismutase (SOD) and catalase (CAT) in mice brains.

Studies have demonstrated that naringin inhibits lipid peroxidation and nitrosative processes by reducing levels of ROS and nitrogen species [44]. Finally, the extract of *Cirsium japonicum* at doses of 200 and 400 mg/kg has shown the ability to reduce immobility time on FST in a similar manner to that of 5 mg/kg of the antidepressant imipramine. A major component of this plant is the flavonoid luteolin, which at doses of 5 and 10 mg/kg produced a similar effect to that of the complete extract, likely through a positive modulating effect on the $GABA_A$ receptor complex. This was proven in an *in vitro* study where extracts of both *Cirsium japonicum* and luteolin increased Cl^- influx in an effect impeded by pretreatment with bicuculline, a competitive $GABA_A$ receptor antagonist [45].

The varied mechanisms seen in flavonoids make them an important object of study, especially in the search for side effect-free treatments that can compromise their effectiveness or produce toxicity by interacting with other medications or food. This is another area of research that remains to be explored.

5. Flavonoids with anxiolytic effects

A particularly important fact concerning the potency of the biological activity of plants is that it depends on several factors, for instance, the part of the plant used, the region where it is gathered, the season, and harvesting time, among others [46]. For example, in male mice evaluated by HBT and EPM, a single dose of 100 mg/kg i.p. of the methanolic extract of inflorescences of *Tilia americana* var. mexicana collected in Morelia, Mexico, produced a more effective anxiolytic effect than those gathered in Honey, Puebla, though the leaves collected in Honey were more effective than those from Morelia or Santa María Ahuacatitlan, Mexico. These three Mexican states are located at different elevations with distinct humidity and soil types. That study quantified quercetin, rutin, and isoquercitrin in the inflorescences and leaves, determining that the concentrations of these substances differed with the part of the plant used and the collection area [46]. It also tested several standard commercial flavonoids: kaempferol (10 mg/kg), quercetin (20 mg/kg), astragalin (10 mg/kg), isoquercitrin (2 mg/kg), quercetin (10 mg/kg), and rutin (15.7 mg/kg), and a mixture of flavonoids (MIX) composed of quercetin 20 mg/kg, rutin 15.7 mg/kg, and isoquercitrin 2 mg/kg and quercetin (20 mg/kg). Results showed that a mixture of quercitin (20 mg/kg), rutin (15.70 mg/kg), and isoquercitrin (2 mg/kg) produced an anxiolytic effect in male mice tested in HBT and EPM [46] by reducing the number of head-dippings but increasing the time spent in the open arms, respectively. Finally, upon testing the anxiolytic effect of the methanolic extract of *Tilia americana* var. mexicana, those authors found that this produced an effect in EPM through the participation of GABA/BDZ (flumazenil 5 mg/kg) and $5HT_{1A}$ serotonergic receptors (WAY 100635 0.5 mg/kg), though they were not involved in the anxiolytic effect on HBT [46].

Another flavonoid known to have anxiolytic effects is formononetin, an active metabolite of traditional Chinese medicine red clover (*Trifolium pratense L.).* Wang et al. [47] observed that administering 25 mg/kg of this metabolite to male mice once daily for 8 days blocked the anxiogenic effect on the open field test (OFT) produced by administering Freund's complete adjuvant (CFA), reduced the time spent and distance traveled in the central area, and decreased the time spent in the open arms of EPM [47]. Formononetin did not modify behavior compared to the control group on either test, indicating that it demonstrated an anxiolytic effect. However, it seems that these results should be understood as a neuroprotective effect more than an anxiolytic one, at least under those study conditions. The notion of a neuroprotector effect is supported by the fact that the study found that formononetin attenuated inflammation and neuronal hyperexcitability by inhibiting NMDA receptors and the CREB signaling pathway in the basolateral amygdala (BLA) [47].

Other anxiolytic mechanisms of action seen in flavonoids are dopaminergic in nature. Theaflavins, for example, increased dopamine (DA) turnover to induce activation of the dopaminergic system in the frontal cortex in male mice in EPM and LDB [48], while chrysin at 2 and 4 mg/kg produced an anxiolytic effect in rats at 12 weeks postovariectomy on LDB by increasing the time spent in the light compartment. Those findings resembled the effect of diazepam. At doses of 1, 2, and 4 mg/kg, this flavonoid increased the frequency of entries into, and the time spent in, the open arms of EPM partially through action on $GABA_A$ receptors (pre-treatment with 1 mg/kg picrotoxin) [49]. On the other hand, neurosteroids and the serotonergic system have also been implicated in the anxiolytic effect of flavonoids, as in the case of puerarin, which increased 5-HT and allopregnanolone levels in the prefrontal cortex and hippocampus in male rats. These results have been associated with the finding that puerarin increased the time spent in the open arms and the percentage of entries into the open arms of EPM, whereas on the VCT test, it produced an increase in the number of shocks received. In both cases, the effect was similar to that of sertraline, which was used as a positive control drug to generate an anxiolytic effect on both tests [50].

In an animal model of surgically-induced menopause, genistein at 0.09 and 0.12 mg/kg, s.c., for seven consecutive days, or the same treatment regimen but with 17β-estradiol, increased the time spent in, and the percentage and frequency of entries into, the open arms of EPM. These effects were caused by activation of the β-estrogenic receptor (ERβ) since pretreatment with tamoxifen (5 mg/kg, an ERβ antagonist) blocked the anxiolytic effect. Also, genistein and 17β-estradiol increased the frequency of rearing and grooming behaviors on the locomotor activity test (LAT), associated with an anxiety-reducing effect manifested in EPM [51]. Genistein tested at doses of 0.25, 0.5, and 1 mg/kg increased the time spent in, and the frequency of exploration of, the light compartment of LDB, while doses of 0.5 and 1 mg/kg increased rearing frequency, and 1 mg/kg increased grooming time. Those studies used rats at 12 weeks postovariectomy [52]. The authors suggest that "genistein is considered a phytoestrogen that acts in a dose-dependent manner with a broader margin of safety at anxiolytic doses. However, more studies are required to take advantage of its potential therapeutic anxiolytic effects" [51].

In a distinct approach, a post-traumatic stress disorder (PTSD) model used a chamber with a grid floor connected to a system that delivered foot shocks, exposing rats to 5 shocks per day. There, an increase in the contextual freezing time on days 7, 14, and 21 indicated the induction of anxiety-like behaviors. The time spent in freezing behavior was calculated with the shock-administering system turned off. In that study, genistein at 4 and 8 mg/kg i.p. administered to male rats from day 7 reduced freezing time at 7, 14, and 21 days. Interestingly, only the 8-mg/kg dose returned freezing times to control levels on day 21 [53]. The stressed rats were also tested in EPM, where they spent less time in the open arms, indicating an anxiety-like effect that was reverted by administering 4 and 8 mg/kg of genistein. This reduced anxiety-like behavior in the stressed rats occurred in association with enhanced tryptophan hydroxylase (TPH) and 5-HT levels, but also promoted the

5-HT receptor-related CaMKII/CREB signaling pathway in the amygdala [53], likely reflecting the fact that the amygdala receives serotonergic projections from the raphe, two brain structures to which emotional valence and 5-HT synthesis, respectively, are attributed [54].

A study evaluated the pharmacokinetic profile of 6-methoxyflavanone and calculated the K_P value (*i.e.*, the tissue-to-serum partition coefficient). Molecules with K_P values >0.30 are thought to be readily distributed in the brain [55]. That study determined that 30 min postadministration of a 30-mg/kg i.p. dose, the 6-methoxyflavanone had crossed the blood-brain barrier (BBB) to reach the amygdala with K_p = 0.47, and the cerebral cortex with K_p = 0.437. These two cerebral structures are known to be involved in the neurobiology of anxiety [56], so these properties were associated with the anxiolytic effect of 6-methoxyflavanone in male and female mice in EPM at doses of 10, 30, and 50 mg/kg, and on the staircase test (ScT). In this model, the lower frequency of rearings, but no reduction in the steps climbed in a 3-min period, was interpreted as indications of an anxiolytic effect [45]. Those authors verified that 6-methoxyflavanone produced its effect by activating $GABA_A$ receptors with the α2-subunit, perhaps in the amygdala and brain cortex, since pretreatment with PTZ blocked this anxiolytic effect in EPM and on ScT [56].

Another flavonoid with anxiolytic effects is rutin at doses of 300 and 562 mg/kg, i.p., or 16 nmol/site, in the basolateral amygdala of male rats tested in EPM. This involves partial GABAergic neurotransmission that was not associated with BDZ binding in the $GABA_A$ receptors [57]. Finally, viscosine administered to male mice assessed in EPM and LDB was seen to exert its action through the α1β2γ2L and α2β2γ2L modulates of the $GABA_A$ receptors at a site distinct from the one classically associated with benzodiazepine [58].

6. Alkaloids with antidepressant activity

Alkaloids purified from crude acid-base extracts have diverse chemical structures. They may contain one or more nitrogen atom(s) (in the heterocyclic ring) in the form of salt [59]. Pseudoalkaloids that possess nitrogen exist. They are not synthesized from amino acids, but by nitrogen transfer in the form of ammonia to a compound of terpenic origin, steroids, polyketides, monosaccharides, or fatty acids [59].

The alkaloid berberine (50 mg/kg, i.p.) decreased immobility but increased climbing behavior on FST; results are considered to reflect an antidepressant-like effect in rats after abstinence from repeated morphine administration [59]. Chronic treatment with the extract of *Annona cherimola* produced antidepressant-like effects in tests of mice on FST. *A. cherimola* contains mainly the alkaloids 1,2-dimethoxy-5,6,6a,7-tetrahydro-4H-dibenzoquinoline-3,8,9,10-tetraol, anonaine, liriodenine, and Nornuciferine, which are likely responsible for the increase in 5-HT and DA [60].

In another work, the alkaloid derivatives of the β-carbolines (harmane 5, 10, and 15 mg/kg, norharmane 2.5, 10, and 15 mg/kg, and harmine 5, 10, and 15 mg/kg, all i.p.) showed antidepressant effects in mice that were dose-dependent, suggesting that the effect occurs through an inverse agonist mechanism of the benzodiazepine receptors due to flumazenil antagonism (5 mg/kg, i.p.) [61]. In addition, anhedonia was reversed in rats subjected to the CUMS model after harmine treatment at 15 mg/kg/day for 7 days. They showed increased adrenal gland weight, ACTH levels, and BNDF protein levels produced by the CUMS [62]. Treatment for 14 days with harmine (5, 10, and 15 mg/kg) and imipramine (10, 20, and 30 mg/kg) in rats subjected to FST produced antidepressant-like effects, while harmine (10 and 15 mg/kg), but not imipramine, increased BDNF protein levels in the hippocampus of rats [62]. These results indicate that the main mechanism involved in harmine's antidepressant effect is an increase in hippocampal BDNF, though this may be dependent on treatment time and the precise region of the hippocampus.

An infusion of harman (1-methyl-beta-carboline) into the hippocampus of rats, or through systemic administration, increased the concentration of 5-HT [63]. In addition, metabolite levels of 5-HT degradation decreased dose-dependently, probably due to inhibition of MAO-A [63]. Another study showed that harman bonds to type 5-HT_{2A} serotonergic receptors but shows no affinity to dopaminergic or BZ receptors [64]. Injections of 2.5 and 10 mg/kg of harmane in rats under fear conditioning have been shown to increase plasma ACTH, corticosterone, 5-HT, and NA levels in limbic system structures. These results suggest that harman can modulate behavioral alterations, brain neurochemistry, and neuroendocrine functions through a mechanism that inhibits MAO-A [65].

Subchronic, oral administration for 21 days of the lyophilized extract of *Rhazya stricta* and alkaloid fractions (akuammidine, rhaziminine, and tetrahydrosecamine) to male rats inhibited the activity of the MAO-B enzyme, a mechanism through which the antidepressant-like effect may occur [66]. Another alkaloid in the *Mitragyna speciosa* plant has shown antidepressant effects. Administered to mice at doses of 10 and 30 mg/kg, i.p., mitragynine decreased immobility time on then TST and FST [67] and the release of corticosterone. Mitragynine's effect appears to be mediated through the neuroendocrine HPA (hypothalamus-adrenal-pituitary) axis [67].

Punarnavine administered at doses of 20 and 40 mg/kg, v.o., for 14 days decreased immobility on FST, MAO-A activity, and corticosterone levels in both stressed and unstressed mice [68], while treatment with evodiamine at 10 and 20 mg/kg in rats exposed to CUMS reversed the decrease in their preference for sugared water and immobility time on FST, but increased 5-HT and NA levels and the protein expression of BNDF in the hippocampus. However, it reduced corticosterone levels, suggesting that it likely modulates monoamines and BDNF-TrkB signaling in the hippocampus [69]. Chronic administration of piperine in rats at 5, 10, and 20 mg/kg has shown antidepressant-like effects on FST, probably due to a serotonergic mechanism [70]. At a dose of 30 mg/kg, protopine produced an antidepressant effect on TST in mice, perhaps by inhibiting the 5-HT and NA transporters, since *in vitro* studies have reported that it produces an inhibitory effect on these elements [71].

Because alkaloids have powerful antidepressant effects, many are used in clinical practice with effective therapeutic results. Preclinical studies have clearly demonstrated the antidepressant effects of alkaloids, but evidence of their mechanisms of action is still deficient or unclear. Alkaloids isolated from plants are an option for treating depression, but more studies are needed at the preclinical level to evaluate their potency, efficacy, and safety before they can be incorporated into clinical practice.

7. Alkaloids with anxiolytic effect

The alkaloids gelsemine, koumine, and gelsevirine exerted anxiolytic effects in single doses of 2 and 10 mg/kg in mice in EPM and LDB [72]. Gelsemine in low doses (10^{-6} M and 10^{-14} M) administered to male rats for 7 days also showed anxiolytic effects in EPM [73]. Koumine has shown this effect on VCT in mice at doses of 0.167, 0.5, or 1.5 mg/kg [74]. Other reports indicate that the decoction of the African peach root (*Nauclea latifolia*) injected intraperitoneally in mice produces dose-dependent anxiolytic-like effects (16, 40, 80, and 160 mg/kg) in EPM. Its effect has been attributed to isoquinoline-type alkaloids [75], but no reports have yet substantiated this claim. One study reported that the isoquinoline alkaloid berberine hydrochloride has both antipsychotic and anxiolytic properties. In this regard, studies have shown that a dose of 100 mg/kg/day produces anxiolytic effects and can modulate the gratifying effects induced by methamphetamine in rats [76].

The aqueous extract of *Eschscholzia californica* Cham (200 mg/kg, p.o.) has shown anxiolytic-like effects on the LDB test in mice that have been attributed to action on $GABA_A$ receptors [77]. Administration of the aqueous extract of the stem of *Uncaria rhynchophylla* (200 mg/kg), which contains the alkaloid rhynchophylline, in a single dose, or for 7 days, produced an anxiolytic effect in EPM by acting on the $5\text{-}HT_{1A}$ receptor [78]. Another example has been implicated to alkaloids with anxiolytic effects were the hydroethanolic extract of *Davilla rugosa* produced anxiolytic-like effects in EPM when administered to rats at 15 mg/kg [79]. Two other plants that contain alkaloids with anxiolytic effects (erythravine and 11a-hydroxy-eritravine) are *Erythrina velutina and Erythrina mulungu.* A study in mice showed that chronic administration (23–26 days) of the hydroalcoholic extract of the stem of *E. velutina* at 100 mg/kg produced an anxiolytic effect in EPM [80], while acute treatment with 200 mg/kg of *E. mulungu* showed an anxiolytic response in LDB comparable to that of diazepam [81]. Nevertheless, in this study did not identify the content or type of alkaloids in these extracts.

Turning to the species Magnolia (*Magnolia spp.*), we find that at least four anxiolytic components have been identified: honokiol, 4-O-methylhonokiol, magnolol, and obovatol. Administering honokiol (1 mg/kg) for 7 days had an anxiolytic-like effect on mice tested in EPM with results similar to those of diazepam [82]. That treatment increased the activity of the enzyme glutamic acid decarboxylase (GAD-subtype 65) in the hippocampus, but not the cortex of the mice brains. This, in turn, increased the release of GABA and reduced anxiety behavior. GAD65 is located on the terminal nerve and regulates the release of GABA to the synaptic cleft [83]. On this topic, there are reports that GAD65-deficient mice show higher anxiety levels [83]. Administering 4-O-methylhonokiol (0.1, 0.2, and 0.5 mg/kg) to mice in a single dose or during 7 days produced anxiolytic effects in EPM through the benzodiazepine site by binding to the $GABA_A$ receptor [84]. This is similar to observations of obovatol at doses of 0.2, 0.5, and 1 mg/kg [85]. In addition, an increase in the expression of the $GABA_A$ receptor $\alpha 1$ subunit [84] and of the $\alpha 1$ subunit in the amygdala and Cl (−) currents was observed [85]. The diterpene alkaloid songorine has shown anxiolytic effects when male mice were tested on VCT at a dose of 0.25 mg/kg [29], revealing an effect similar to that of phenazepam.

Numerous reports attribute anxiolytic activity to a broad range of plants. However, isolating and identifying the alkaloids responsible for this activity have not advanced substantially. Preclinical reports point to a common mechanism of action that modulates the GABAergic and serotonergic systems. The data described here justifies the need to conduct preclinical and clinical studies using alkaloids as alternative treatments for some anxiety disorders.

8. Sterols with anxiolytic and antidepressant effects

Plants synthesize a class of sterols called phytosterols, whose chemical structure is similar to that of cholesterol. Phytosterols are found in nuts, vegetable oils, cereals, fruits, vegetables, and various plants [86]. Some 40 different types have been identified, including β-sitosterol, campesterol, fucosterol, and stigmasterol. Due to their lipidic nature and glycosylated forms, they are able to cross the blood-brain barrier and impact the CNS [87]. Trevisan et al. [88] suggest that α-spinasterol has the ability to cross the blood-brain barrier and exert an antagonistic effect on the transient potential receptor V1 (TRPV1). When these receptors are expressed in various areas of the brain—prefrontal cortex, amygdala, hypothalamus, and hippocampus—their activation augments the release of glutamate and, consequently, that of GABA, DA, or other catecholamines [89]. This fact involved TRPV1 receptors in the mechanism underlying the etiology of depression and anxiety. This was corroborated by Socała and Wlaź [90] by administering (1 and 2 mg/kg, i.p.) α-spinasterol to male mice and testing them on FST. Their results suggest an antidepressant effect. Also, intracerebroventricular (i.c.v.) coadministration of 50 μg of the TRPV1 receptor antagonist capsazepine/mouse with an ineffective dose of 0.5 mg/kg, i.p., of α-spinasterol, also reduced immobility time on FST, indicating the involvement of TRPV1 in the neurobiology of depression. However, α-spinasterol itself (0.5, 1, and 2 mg/kg) was unable to produce anxiolytic-like effects in EPM or LDB. In this sense, TRPV1-knockout mice manifested less anxiety behavior on the same tests [91]. Socała and Wlaź [90] proposed that α-spinasterol may be able to activate CB1 receptors with greater affinity because those neurons coexpress these receptors in various brain structures whose activation could activate TRPV1 receptors simultaneously to block their possible anxiolytic effects. In another work, administering fucosterol (10, 20, 30, or 40 mg/kg, v.o.) to male mice produced antidepressant effects on FST and TST, with the 20 and 30 mg/kg doses achieving an effect of comparable efficacy to 20 mg/kg of fluoxetine, a standard dose in humans [92]. Those doses also exerted an acute effect that increased BDNF levels in the hippocampus, a limbic structure involved in mood regulation. Fucosterol also blocked the decrease in 5-HT, 5-HTIIA, and NA levels in mice brains generated by the stress of FST. The effect of fucosterol on that test was similar to that of the positive control drug, but it was unable to prevent the reduction of DA, another factor caused by FST. These findings suggest that the antidepressant mechanism is mediated by increasing monoamines and reducing the rate of 5-HT metabolism. Fucosterol did not modify either motor or exploratory activity and showed no neurotoxic effects [92]. Similar results were found when administering β-sitosterol at 10, 20, and 30 mg/kg for 7 days. In that case, 30 mg/kg exerted effects similar to those of 20 mg/kg of fluoxetine on FST and TST. Finally, the effects on monoamine levels in mice brains confirm that sterols modify the serotonergic and noradrenergic systems but do not impact the dopaminergic system [93].

Another case involved α- and β-amyrin (αβAMY) isolated from the resin of the stem of *Protium heptaphyllum* plants obtained and identified from hexane-ethyl acetate fractions analyzed by TLC. That process produced 450 mg of αβAMY made up of 67% α- and 33% β-amyrin, which were further purified and tested on FST. Administering 2.5 and 5 mg/kg of αβAMY via i.p. or p.o. decreased immobility time, but the most effective treatment was the 2.5-mg/kg dose via the p.o. route. However, the effects produced by this route were similar to those of imipramine at 30 and 10 mg/kg. Imipramine is a tricyclic antidepressant (TCA) that blocks reuptake of both serotonin and norepinephrine. In addition, a pharmacological synergism between 1 or 2.5 mg/kg of αβAMY and 10 mg/kg of imipramine was observed, but not between 2.5 mg/kg of αβAMY and 4 mg/kg of paroxetine (SSRIs). These effects were blocked by pretreatment with 2 mg/kg of reserpine, an inhibitor of the vesicular catecholamine transporter that facilitates vesicular storage. This result suggests a possible mechanism of action through activation of the noradrenergic system [94]. The base structure that cholesterol and sterols share allows the latter to exert actions at the level of the CNS, as in the case of cholesterol. Cholesterol is a vital substance for neurons because it is required for vesicle transport and neurotransmitter release and as a precursor to neurosteroids. It is also implicated in synaptic plasticity in relation to the formation of new synapses. For these reasons, studying sterols and their mechanisms of action on the CNS is extremely important because of the anxiolytic and/or antidepressant effects they exert.

9. Final comments and conclusion

This broad review constitutes a significant contribution to our understanding of the mechanisms of action that allow plants to produce antidepressant and anxiolytic effects (see **Figure 1** for a summary). However, most of the studies reviewed were conducted with mice, due to the low yields achieved when isolating the metabolites of plant extracts [95], which limit the amount of testing that can be done. Another

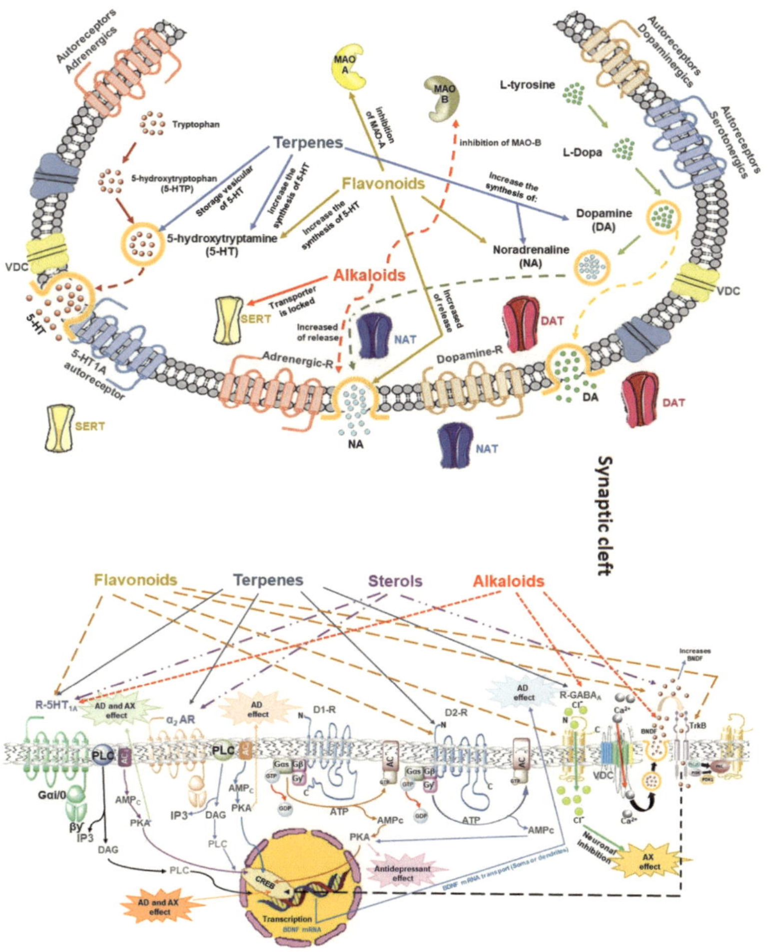

Figure 1.

Principal mechanisms of action of flavonoids, terpenes, sterols, and alkaloids with antidepressant and anxiolytic properties. DAG: diacylglycerol; IP3: inositol triphosphate; AMPC: adenosine monophosphate 3; PKA: protein kinase A; PLC: phospholipase C; AC: adenylyl cyclase; ATP: adenosine triphosphate; GDP: guanosin trifosfato; VDC: canal dependiente de voltaje; BNDF: factor neurotrófico derivado del cerebro; TrkB: tropomyosin receptor kinase B; Ca^{2+}: calcium ion; Cl^{-}: chloride ion; R-5HT_{1A}: 5HT_{1A} receptor; α_2AR: alpha 2-adrenergic receptor; D1-R: dopamine receptor D1; D2-R: dopamine receptor D2; DAT: dopamine transporter; NAT: noradrenaline transporter; SERT: serotonin transporter; MAO-A: monoamine oxidase A; MAO-B: monoamine oxidase B; AD: antidepressant; AX: anxiolytic.

concern is that some infusions or extracts used as household remedies lose their antidepressant or anxiolytic effects when fractioned [96]. These findings indicate that in some cases it may be necessary to keep the metabolites together at the concentrations present in the original infusion or extract that has a proven therapeutic effect. As explained herein, some metabolites share pharmacological targets, which explains why they lose their effect when separated and emphasizes the importance of using standardized extracts with demonstrated therapeutic effects in animal and human studies [97, 98]. Unfortunately, very few clinical studies have evaluated the potential antidepressant or anxiolytic effects of isolated metabolites, so a great deal of work remains to be done.

Several observations suggest that active metabolites share the mechanism of action of antidepressant and anxiolytic drugs like SSRIs, SNRIs, MAOIs, DDNRI, and BZDs, but we should emphasize that some metabolites—at least in preclinical studies—produced better effects than conventional drugs, even at lower doses, while others presented a pharmacological synergism between both types at suboptimal doses that improved the effects exerted separately at higher doses. A second shared characteristic is that they contain active stereoisomers and probably, some metabolites, once metabolized, could become more active. This encourages us to consider a significant number of substances with anxiolytic and/or antidepressant pharmacological profiles and invites us to take on the challenge of evaluating their pharmacokinetics, pharmacodynamics, and safety.

In conclusion, terpenes, flavonoids, alkaloids, and sterols share mechanisms of action that include activation of the critical enzyme for catecholamine synthesis (e.g., tyrosine hydroxylase) or the inhibition of their limiting enzymes, MAO-A and MAO-B, and transporters, thus stimulating the vesicular storage monoamine and the release of neurotransmitters toward the synaptic cleft. Finally, they can prevent the production of ROS and inhibit NO synthesis and, further downstream, interact with the 5-HT_{1A}, 5-HT_{2A}, D1, D2, $GABA_A$ receptors, and $\alpha 1$, $\alpha 2$, β-adrenoceptors that contribute to stimulating PKA. One consequence is that CREB increases BDNF levels, which foster the appearance of dendritic contacts that improve cerebral neurotransmission and modulate the emotions.

10. Perspective

This chapter discusses the efficacy of some plant metabolites in treating anxiety and depression disorders, as demonstrated in preclinical studies. In the future, this option for treating such disorders will allow us to reduce treatment costs and moderate the side effects produced by drugs currently in use. However, our review also points out that few clinical studies have focused on the pharmacokinetic and pharmacodynamic processes involving metabolites that would permit the safe use of these extracts. Despite this, research has shown that traditional medicine, especially forms that use medicinal plants that have been passed down through several generations, constitutes an important alternative for health care.

Acknowledgements

The third author received (Ramos-Molina Ana Raquel) fellowships from Consejo Nacional de Ciencia y Tecnología (CONACyT) for postgraduate studies in Science and Technology (Reg. 631048).

Author details

Rosa Isela García-Ríos[1]*, Armando Mora-Pérez[1], Ana Raquel Ramos-Molina[2] and Cesar Soria-Fregozo[1]

1 Laboratory of Psychobiology, University Center of Los Lagos, University of Guadalajara, Lagos de Moreno, Jalisco, Mexico

2 University Center of Los Lagos, University of Guadalajara, Lagos de Moreno, Jalisco, Mexico

*Address all correspondence to: rosai_garios@yahoo.com

References

[1] Global Burden of Disease (GBD). Available from: https://vizhub.healthdata.org/gbd-compare/. [Accessed: 05 August 2019]

[2] Depression and Other Common Mental Disorders: Global Health Estimates. Geneva: World Health Organization; 2017. Licence: CC BY-NC-SA 3.0 IGO

[3] Anxiety.org. [Internet] 2019. Available from: https://www.anxiety.org/what-is-anxiety [Accessed: 05 August 2019]

[4] Rakofsky JJ, Holtzheimer PE, Nemeroff CB. Emerging targets for antidepressant therapies. Current Opinion in Chemical Biology. 2009; **13**(3):291-302

[5] Trivedi MH, Rush AJ, Wisniewski SR, Nierenberg AA, Warden D, Ritz L, et al. Evaluation of outcomes with citalopram for depression using measurement-based care in STAR*D: Implications for clinical practice. The American Journal of Psychiatry. 2006;**163**(1):28-40

[6] Rush AJ, Trivedi MH, Wisniewski SR, Stewart JW, Nierenberg AA, Thase ME, et al. Bupropion-SR, sertraline, or venlafaxine-XR after failure of SSRIs for depression. The New England Journal of Medicine. 2006;**354**(12):1231-1242

[7] Papakostas GI. Tolerability of modern antidepressants. The Journal of Clinical Psychiatry. 2008;**69**(E1):8-13

[8] Griebel G, Holmes A. 50 years of hurdles and hope in anxiolytic drug discovery. Nature Reviews. Drug Discovery. 2013;**12**:667-687

[9] New WHO guidelines to promote proper use of alternative medicines [Internet] 2004. Available from: https://www.who.int/mediacentre/news/releases/2004/pr44/en/. WHO Guidelines: Developing Information on Proper Use of Traditional, Complementary and Alternative Medicine [pdf 3.1Mb] [Accessed: 01 July 2019]

[10] WHO Traditional Medicine Strategy: 2014–2023. Hong Kong SAR, China: Organización Mundial de la Salud; 2013. ISBN: 978 92 4 350609 8 (Clasificación NLM: WB 55)

[11] López-Rubalcava C, Estrada-Camarena E. Mexican medicinal plants with anxiolytic or antidepressant activity: Focus on preclinical research. Journal of Ethnopharmacology. 2016; **186**:377-391

[12] Fajemiroye JO, da Silva DM, de Oliveira DR, Costa EA. Treatment of anxiety and depression: Medicinal plants in retrospect. Fundamental & Clinical Pharmacology. 2016;**30**(3): 198-215

[13] Lundstrom K, Pham HT, Dinh LD. Interaction of plant extracts with central nervous system receptors. Medicines (Basel). 2017;**4**(1):1-13

[14] Arnason JT, Catling PM, Small E, Dang PT, Lambert JDH. Biodiversity & health: Focusing research to policy. In: Proceeding of the International Symposium, NRC Research Press, Canada. 2005

[15] Abdelhalim A, Karim N, Chebib M, Aburjai T, Khan I, Johnston GA, et al. Antidepressant, anxiolytic and antinociceptive activities of constituents from *Rosmarinus officinalis*. Journal of Pharmacy & Pharmaceutical Sciences. 2015;**18**(4):448-459

[16] Machado DG, Cunha MP, Neis VB, Balen GO, Colla A, Bettio LE, et al. Antidepressant-like effects of fractions, essential oil, carnosol and betulinic acid

isolated from *Rosmarinus officinalis* L. Food Chemistry. 2013;**136**(2):999-1005

[17] Khan I, Karim N, Ahmad W, Abdelhalim A, Chebib M. GABA-A receptor modulation and anticonvulsant, anxiolytic, and antidepressant activities of constituents from *Artemisia indica* Linn. Evidence-based Complementary and Alternative Medicine. 2016;**1215393**

[18] Machado DG, Neis VB, Balen GO, Colla A, Cunha MP, Dalmarco JB, et al. Antidepressant-like effect of ursolic acid isolated from *Rosmarinus officinalis* L. in mice: Evidence for the involvement of the dopaminergic system. Pharmacology, Biochemistry, and Behavior. 2012;**103**(2):204-211

[19] Colla AR, Oliveira A, Pazini FL, Rosa JM, Manosso LM, Cunha MP, et al. Serotonergic and noradrenergic systems are implicated in the antidepressant-like effect of ursolic acid in mice. Pharmacology, Biochemistry, and Behavior. 2014;**124**:108-116

[20] Saeid A-M, Zohre K, Rahim T-F. The antidepressant-like effects of *Origanum majorana* essential oil on mice through monoaminergic modulation using the forced swimming test. Journal of Traditional and Complementary Medicine. DOI: 10.1016/j.jtcme.2019.01.003. [Accessed: 14 January 2019] in press

[21] Coelho V, Mazzardo-Martins L, Martins DF, Santos AR, da Silva Brum LF, Picada JN, et al. Neurobehavioral and genotoxic evaluation of (−)-linalool in mice. Journal of Natural Medicines. 2013; **67**(4):876-880

[22] Guzmán-Gutiérrez SL, Bonilla-Jaime H, Gómez-Cansino R, Reyes-Chilpa R. Linalool and β-pinene exert their antidepressant-like activity through the monoaminergic pathway. Life Sciences. 2015;**128**:24-29

[23] Gomes PB, Feitosa ML, Silva MI, Noronha EC, Moura BA, Venâncio ET, et al. Anxiolytic-like effect of the monoterpene 1,4-cineole in mice. Pharmacology, Biochemistry, and Behavior. 2010;**96**(3):287-293

[24] González-Trujano ME, Hernández-Sánchez LY, Muñoz Ocotero V, Dorazco-González A, Guevara Fefer P, Aguirre-Hernández E. Pharmacological evaluation of the anxiolytic-like effects of *Lippia graveolens* and bioactive compounds. Pharmaceutical Biology. 2017;**55**(1):1569-1576

[25] Moreira MR, Salvadori MG, de Almeida AA, de Sousa DP, Jordán J, Satyal P, et al. Anxiolytic-like effects and mechanism of (−)-myrtenol: A monoterpene alcohol. Neuroscience Letters. 2014;**579**:119-124

[26] Costa CA, Cury TC, Cassettari BO, Takahira RK, Flório JC, Costa M. *Citrus aurantium* L. essential oil exhibits anxiolytic-like activity mediated by 5-HT(1A)-receptors and reduces cholesterol after repeated oral treatment. BMC Complement and Alternative Medicine. 2013;**13**:42

[27] Zhang N, Yao L. Anxiolytic effect of essential oils and their constituents: A review. Journal of Agricultural and Food Chemistry. 2019. DOI: 10.1021/acs.jafc.9b00433 in press

[28] Souto-Maior FN, de Carvalho FL, de Morais LC, Netto SM, de Sousa DP, de Almeida RN. Anxiolytic-like effects of inhaled linalool oxide in experimental mouse anxiety models. Pharmacology, Biochemistry, and Behavior. 2011; **100**(2):259-263

[29] Nesterova YV, Povet'eva TN, Suslov NI, Shults EE, Ziuz'kov GN, Aksinenko SG, et al. Anxiolytic activity of diterpene alkaloid songorine. Bulletin of Experimental Biology and Medicine. 2015;**159**(5):620-622

[30] German-Ponciano LJ, Rosas-Sánchez GU, Rivadeneyra-Domínguez E, Rodríguez-Landa JF. Advances in the preclinical study of some flavonoids as potential antidepressant agents. Scientifica. 2018; **1**:2963565

[31] Liu LX, Chen WF, Xie JX, Wong MS. Neuroprotective effects of genistein on dopaminergic neurons in the mice model of Parkinson's disease. Neuroscience Research. 2008;**60**: 156-161

[32] Tsai TH. Concurrent measurement of unbound genistein in the blood, brain and bile of anesthetized rats using microdialysis and its pharmacokinetic application. Journal of Chromatography. A. 2005;**1073**(1–2):317-322

[33] Hu P, Ma L, Wang YG, Ye F, Wang C, Zhou WH, et al. Genistein, a dietary soy isoflavone, exerts antidepressant-like effects in mice: Involvement of serotonergic system. Neurochemistry International. 2017; **108**:426-435

[34] Kageyama A, Sakakibara H, Zhou W, Yoshioka M, Ohsumi M, Shimoi K, et al. Genistein regulated serotonergic activity in the hippocampus of ovariectomized rats under forced swimming stress. Bioscience, Biotechnology, and Biochemistry. 2010;**74**(10):2005-2010

[35] Sapronov NS, Kasakova SB. Effects of synthetic and plant-derived selective modulators of estrogen receptors on depression-like behavior of female rats. Bulletin of Experimental Biology and Medicine. 2008;**146**(1):73-76

[36] Singh V, Chauhan G, Shri R. Anti-depressant like effects of quercetin 4'-O-glucoside from *Allium cepa* via regulation of brain oxidative stress and monoamine levels in mice subjected to unpredictable chronic mild stress. Nutritional Neuroscience. 2019;**1**:1-10

[37] Holzmann I, da Silva LM, Corrêa da Silva JA, Steimbach VM, de Souza MM. Antidepressant-like effect of quercetin in bulbectomized mice and involvement of the antioxidant defenses, and the glutamatergic and oxidonitrergic pathways. Pharmacology Biochemistry and Behavior. 2015;**136**:55-63

[38] Lindqvist D, Dhabhar FS, James SJ, Hough CM, Jain FA, Bersani FS, et al. Oxidative stress, inflammation and treatment response in major depression. Psychoneuroendocrinology. 2017;**76**: 197-205

[39] Filho CB, Jesse CR, Donato F, Del Fabbro L, Gomes de Gomes M, Rossito Goes AT, et al. Chrysin promotes attenuation of depressive-like behavior and hippocampal dysfunction resulting from olfactory bulbectomy in mice. Chemico-Biological Interactions. 2016; **260**:154-162

[40] Wang Y, Wang B, Lu J, Shi H, Gong S, Wang Y, et al. Fisetin provides antidepressant effects by activating the tropomyosin receptor kinase B signal pathway in mice. Journal of Neurochemistry. 2017;**143**(5):561-568

[41] Ren Z, Yan P, Zhu L, Yang H, Zhao Y, Kirby BP, et al. Dihydromyricetin exerts a rapid antidepressant-like effect in association with enhancement of BDNF expression and inhibition of neuroinflammation. Psychopharmacology. 2018;**235**(1): 233-244

[42] Donato F, de Gomes MG, Goes AT, Filho CB, Del Fabbro L, Antunes MS, et al. Hesperidin exerts antidepressant-like effects in acute and chronic treatments in mice: Possible role of l-arginine-NO-cGMP pathway and BDNF levels. Brain Research Bulletin. 2014; **104**:19-26

[43] Zhang R, Ma Z, Liu K, Li Y, Liu D, Xu L, et al. Baicalin exerts antidepressant effects through

Akt/FOXG1 pathway promoting neuronal differentiation and survival. Life Sciences. 2019;**15**(221):241-248

[44] Ben-Azu B, Nwoke EE, Aderibigbe AO, Omogbiya IA, Ajayi AM, Olonode ET, et al. Possible neuroprotective mechanisms of action involved in the neurobehavioral property of naringin in mice. Biomedicine & Pharmacotherapy. 2019; **109**:536-546

[45] de la Peña JB, Kim CA, Lee HL, Yoon SY, Kim HJ, Hong EY, et al. Luteolin mediates the antidepressant-like effects of *Cirsium japonicum* in mice, possibly through modulation of the GABAA receptor. Archives of Pharmacal Research. 2014;**37**(2): 263-269

[46] Aguirre-Hernández E, González-Trujano ME, Terrazas T, Herrera Santoyo J, Guevara-Fefer P. Anxiolytic and sedative-like effects of flavonoids from *Tilia americana* var. mexicana: GABAergic and serotonergic participation. Salud Mental. 2001;**39**(1): 37-46

[47] Wang XS, Guan SY, Liu A, Yue J, Hu LN, Zhang K, et al. Anxiolytic effects of formononetin in an inflammatory pain mouse model. Molecular Brain. 2019;**12**(1):36

[48] Kita M, Uchida S, Yamada K, Ano Y. Anxiolytic effects of theaflavins via dopaminergic activation in the frontal cortex. Bioscience, Biotechnology, and Biochemistry. 2019; **83**(6):1157-1162

[49] Rodríguez-Landa JF, Hernández-López F, Cueto-Escobedo J, Herrera-Huerta EV, Rivadeneyra-Domínguez E, Bernal-Morales B, et al. Chrysin (5,7-dihydroxyflavone) exerts anxiolytic-like effects through GABAA receptors in a surgical menopause model in rats. Biomedicine & Pharmacotherapy. 2019; **109**:2387-2395

[50] Qiu ZK, Zhang GH, Zhong DS, He JL, Liu X, Chen JS, et al. Puerarin ameliorated the behavioral deficits induced by chronic stress in rats. Scientific Reports. 2017;**7**(1):6266

[51] Rodríguez-Landa JF, Cueto-Escobedo J, Puga-Olguín A, Rivadeneyra-Domínguez E, Bernal-Morales B, Herrera-Huerta EV, et al. The phytoestrogen genistein produces similar effects as 17β-estradiol on anxiety-like behavior in rats at 12 weeks after ovariectomy. BioMed Research International. 2017;**2017**: 9073816

[52] Rodríguez-Landa JF, Hernández-Figueroa JD, Hernández-Calderón BC, Saavedra M. Anxiolytic-like effect of phytoestrogen genistein in rats with long-term absence of ovarian hormones in the black and white model. Progress in Neuro-Psychopharmacology & Biological Psychiatry. 2009;**33**(2): 367-372

[53] Wu ZM, Ni GL, Shao AM, Cui R. Genistein alleviates anxiety-like behaviors in post-traumatic stress disorder model through enhancing serotonergic transmission in the amygdala. Psychiatry Research. 2017; **255**:287-291

[54] Kelmendi B, Adams TG, Yarnell S, Southwick S, Abdallah CG, Krystal JH. PTSD: From neurobiology to pharmacological treatments. European Journal of Psychotraumatology. 2016; **8**(7):31858

[55] Di L, Kerns EH, Carter GT. Strategies to assess blood-brain barrier penetration. Expert Opinion on Drug Discovery. 2008;**3**(6):677-687

[56] Akbar S, Subhan F, Karim N, Aman U, Ullah S, Shahid M, et al. Characterization of 6-methoxyflavanone as a novel anxiolytic agent: A behavioral and pharmacokinetic approach. European

Journal of Pharmacology. 2017;**801**: 19-27

[57] Hernandez-Leon A, González-Trujano ME, Fernández-Guasti A. The anxiolytic-like effect of rutin in rats involves $GABA_A$ receptors in the basolateral amygdala. Behavioural Pharmacology. 2017;**28**(4): 303-312

[58] Karim N, Irshad S, Khan I, Mohammad A, Anis I, Shah MR, et al. GABA(A) receptor modulation and neuropharmacological activities of viscosine isolated from *Dodonaea viscosa* (Linn). Pharmacology, Biochemistry, and Behavior. 2015;**136**:64-72

[59] Lee B, Sur B, Yeom M, Shim I, Lee H, Hahm DH. Effect of berberine on depression- and anxiety-like behaviors and activation of the noradrenergic system induced by development of morphine dependence in rats. The Korean Journal of Physiology & Pharmacology. 2012;**16**(6):379-386

[60] Martínez-Vázquez M, Estrada-Reyes R, Araujo Escalona AG, Velázquez IL, Martínez-Mota L, Morenod J, et al. Antidepressant-like effects of an alkaloid extract of the aerial parts of *Annona cherimolia* in mice. Journal of Ethnopharmacology. 2012; **139**:164-170

[61] Farzin D, Mansouri N. Antidepressant-like effect of harmane and other β-carbolines in the mouse forced swim test. European Neuropsychopharmacology. 2006;**16**: 324-328

[62] Fortunato JJ, Réus GZ, Kirsch TR, Stringari RB, Fries GR, Kapczinski F, et al. Effects of beta-carboline harmine on behavioral and physiological parameters observed in the chronic mild stress model: Further evidence of antidepressant properties. Brain Research Bulletin. 2010;**81**(4–5): 491-496

[63] Adell A, Biggs TA, Myersb RD. Action of Harman (l-methyl-P-carboline) on the brain: Body temperature and in viva efflux of 5-HT from hippocampus of the rat. Neuropharmacology. 1996;**35**: 1101-1107

[64] Glennon RA, Dukat M, Grella B, Hong S, Costantino L, Teitler M, et al. Binding of b-carbolines and related agents at serotonin (5-HT2 and 5-HT1A), dopamine (D2) and benzodiazepine receptors. Drug and Alcohol Dependence. 2000;**60**:121-132

[65] Smith KL, Ford GK, Jessop DS, Finn DP. Behavioural, neurochemical and neuroendocrine effects of the endogenous β-carboline harmane in fear-conditioned rats. Journal of Psychopharmacology. 2013;**2**:162-170

[66] Ali BH, Bashir AK, Tanira MOM, Medvedev AE, Jarrett N, Sandler M, et al. Effect of extract of *Rhazya stricta*, a traditional medicinal plant, on rat brain tribulin. Pharmacology, Biochemistry, and Behavior. 1998;**59**:671-675

[67] Idayu NF, Hidayata MT, Moklasa MAM, Sharidaa F, Raudzaha ARN, Shamimaa AR, et al. Antidepressant-like effect of mitragynine isolated from *Mitragyna speciosa* Korth in mice model of depression. Phytomedicine. 2011;**18**: 402-407

[68] Dhingra D, Valecha R. Punarivine, an alkaloid isolated from ethanolic extract of *Boerhaavia diffusa* Linn, reverses depression-like behaviour in mice subject to chronic unpredictable mild stress. Indian Journal of Experimental Biology. 2014;**52**:799-807

[69] Jiang ML, Zhang ZX, Li YZ, Wang XH, Yan W, Gong GQ. Antidepressant-like effect of evodiamine on chronic unpredictable mild stress rats. Neuroscience Letters. 2015;**588**:154-158

[70] Wattanathorn J, Chonpathompikunlert P, Muchimapura S, Priprem A, Tankamnerdthai O. Piperine, the potential functional food for mood and cognitive disorders. Food and Chemical Toxicology. 2008;**46**:3106-3110

[71] Xu LF, Chu WJ, Qing XY, Li S, Wang XS, Qing GW, et al. Protopine inhibits serotonin transporter and noradrenaline transporter and has the antidepressant-like effect in mice models. Neuropharmacology. 2006;**50**:934-940

[72] Liu M, Huang HH, Yang J, Su YP, Lin HW, Lin LQ, et al. The active alkaloids of *Gelsemium elegans* Benth., are potent anxiolytics. Psychopharmacology. 2013;**225**(4):839-851

[73] Meyer L, Boujedaini N, Patte-Mensah C, Mensah-Nyagan AG. Pharmacological effect of gelsemine on anxiety-like behavior in rat. Behavioural Brain Research. 2013;**253**:90-94

[74] Chen CJ, Zhong ZF, Xin ZM, Hong LH, Su YP, Yu CX. Koumine exhibits anxiolytic properties without inducing adverse neurological effects on functional observation battery, open-field and Vogel conflict tests in rodents. Journal of Natural Medicines. 2017;**71**(2):397-408

[75] Ngo Bum E, Taiwe GS, Moto FC, et al. Anticonvulsant, anxiolytic, and sedative properties of the roots of *Nauclea latifolia* Smith in mice. Epilepsy & Behavior. 2009;**15**(4):434-440

[76] Alavijeh MM, Vaezi G, Khaksari M, Hojati V. Berberine hydrochloride attenuates voluntary methamphetamine consumption and anxiety-like behaviors via modulation of oxytocin receptors in methamphetamine addicted rats. Physiology & Behavior. 2019;**206**:157-165

[77] Rolland A, Fleurentin J, Lanhers MC, et al. Neurophysiological effects of an extract of *Eschscholzia californica* Cham. (Papaveraceae). Phytotherapy Research. 2001;**15**(5):377-381

[78] Jung JW, Ahn NY, Oh HR, Lee BK, Lee KJ, Kim SY, et al. Anxiolytic effects of the aqueous extract of *Uncaria rhynchophylla*. Journal of Ethnopharmacology. 2006;**108**(2):193-197

[79] Guaraldo L, Chagas DA, Konno AC, et al. Hydroalcoholic extract and fractions of *Davilla rugosa* Poiret: Effects on spontaneous motor activity and elevated plus-maze behavior. Journal of Ethnopharmacology. 2000;**72**(1–2):61-67

[80] Raupp IM, Sereniki A, Virtuoso S, et al. Anxiolytic-like effect of chronic treatment with *Erythrina velutina* extract in the elevated plus-maze test. Journal of Ethnopharmacology. 2008;**118**(2):295-299

[81] Onusic GM, Nogueira RL, Pereira AM, et al. Effect of acute treatment with a water-alcohol extract of *Erythrina mulungu* on anxiety-related responses in rats. Brazilian Journal of Medical and Biological Research. 2002;**35**(4):473-477

[82] Ku TH, Lee YJ, Wang SJ, et al. Effect of honokiol on activity of GAD(65) and GAD(67) in the cortex and hippocampus of mice. Phytomedicine. 2011;**18**(13):1126-1129

[83] Kash SF, Tecott LH, Hodge C, Baekkeskov S. Increased anxiety and altered responses to anxiolytics in mice deficient in the 65-kDa isoform of glutamic acid decarboxylase. Proceedings of the National Academy of Sciences of the United States of America. 1999;**96**(4):1698-1703

[84] Han H, Jung JK, Han SB, et al. Anxiolytic-like effects of 4-Omethylhonokiol isolated from *Magnolia officinalis* through enhancement of GABAergic transmission and chloride influx. Journal of Medicinal Food. 2011;**14**(7–8):724-731

[85] Seo JJ, Lee SH, Lee YS, et al. Anxiolytic-like effects of obovatol isolated from *Magnolia obovata*: Involvement of GABA/benzodiazepine receptors complex. Progress in Neuro-Psychopharmacology & Biological Psychiatry. 2007;**31**(7):1363-1369

[86] Klingberg S, Andersson H, Mulligan A, Bhaniani A, Welch A, Bingham S. Food sources of plant sterols in the EPIC Norfolk population. European Journal of Clinical Nutrition. 2008;**62**:695-703

[87] Tabata RC, Wilson JM, Zwiegers P, Kwok D, Van Kampen JM. Chronic exposure to dietary sterol glucosides is neurotoxic to motor neuronsand induces an ALS-PDC phenotype. NeuroMolecular Medicine. 2008;**10**: 24-39

[88] Trevisan G, Rossato MF, Walker CI, Klafke JZ, Rosa F, Oliveira SM. Identification of the plant steroid alpha-spinasterol as a novel transient receptor potential vanilloid 1 antagonist with antinociceptive properties. The Journal of Pharmacology and Experimental Therapeutics. 2012;**343**(2):258-269

[89] Martins D, Tavares I, Morgado C. Hotheaded: The role of TRPV1 in brain functions. Neuropharmacology. 2014; **85**:151-157

[90] Socała K, Wlaź P. Evaluation of the antidepressant- and anxiolytic-like activity of α-spinasterol, a plant derivative with TRPV1 antagonistic effects, in mice. Behavioural Brain Research. 2016;**5**(303):19-25

[91] Marsch R, Foeller E, Rammes G, Bunck M, Kössl M, Holsboer F, et al. Reduced anxiety, conditioned fear, and hippocampal long-term potentiation in transient receptor potential vanilloid type 1 receptor-deficient mice. The Journal of Neuroscience. 2007;**27**(4): 832-839

[92] Zhen XH, Quan YC, Jiang HY, Wen ZS, Qu YL, Guan LP. Fucosterol, a sterol extracted from *Sargassum fusiforme*, shows antidepressant and anticonvulsant effects. European Journal of Pharmacology. 2015;**768**: 131-138

[93] Zhao D, Zheng L, Qi L, Wang S, Guan L, Xia Y, et al. Structural features and potent antidepressant effects of total sterols and β-sitosterol extracted from *Sargassum horneri*. Marine Drugs. 2016;**14**:123

[94] Aragão GF, Carneiro LM, Junior APF, Vieira LC, Bandeira PN, Lemos TLG, et al. A possible mechanism for anxiolytic and antidepressant effects of alpha- and beta-amyrin from *Protium heptaphyllum* (Aubl.) March. Pharmacology, Biochemistry and Behavior. 2007;**85**(4):827-834

[95] Cassani J, Dorantes-Barrón AM, Novales LM, Real GA, Estrada-Reyes R. Anti-depressant-like effect of kaempferitrin isolated from *Justicia spicigera* Schltdl (Acanthaceae) in two behavior models in mice: Evidence for the involvement of the serotonergic system. Molecules. 2014;**19**(12): 21442-21461

[96] Nogueira E, Rosa GJ, Haraguchi M, Vassilieff VS. Anxiolytic effect *of Rubus brasilensis* in rats and mice. Journal of Ethnopharmacology. 1998;**61**(2): 111-117

[97] Liu R, Ahmed F, Cayer C, Mullally M, Carballo AF, Rojas MO, et al. New botanical anxiolytics for use

in companion animals and humans. The AAPS Journal. 2017;**19**(6):1626-1631

[98] Lima EBC, de Sousa CNS, Meneses LN, E Silva Pereira YF, Matos NCB, de Freitas RB, et al. Involvement of monoaminergic systems in anxiolytic and antidepressive activities of the standardized extract of *Cocos nucifera* L. Journal of Natural Medicines. 2017;**71**(1):227-237

Chapter 6

Neuropharmacology of Anxiety Disorders at Young Age: A Perspective from Preclinical Research

Gabriel Guillén-Ruiz, Blandina Bernal-Morales, César Soria-Fregozo, Emma Virginia Herrera-Huerta, Ana Karen Limón-Vázquez, Margarita Hernández-Mixteco and Abraham Puga-Olguín

Abstract

Anxiety is one of the most common psychopathologies in the general population that often begin early in life; however, research on this disorder during early developmental stages has been poorly explored compared to adults. A better understanding of the anxiety disorder through childhood is essential to develop more effective treatments. This chapter provides a general overview of the usefulness of animal models of childhood anxiety and its neurobiological bases to discuss how the studies on animals meet the several criteria of validity to discover pathophysiological mechanisms of human disorders and new treatments for these conditions. The research methodology for this chapter consisted in using a thesaurus system such as Medical Subject Headings (MeSH) terms of the National Library of Medicine to find original articles in databases as PubMed or Web of Science about preclinical findings related to the neuropharmacology of anxiety before adulthood. The contribution of this chapter is to provide data from preclinical studies which are encouraged to a better comprehension of anxiety at young age.

Keywords: adolescent, anxiety, anxiolytics, animal model, child, rats

1. Introduction

Anxiety is a disorder that can be developed in offspring as a result of aversive life conditions. Some factors in the childhood and adolescence that predispose the development of anxiety disorders include sexual abuse [1], social isolation [2], maternal separation [3], physical abuse, emotional abuse, negligence, and exposure to partner violence [4]. In addition, children who experience multiple types of abuse can suffer exacerbate symptoms of anxiety and comorbidity with depression compared to those who are only exposed to one type of abuse [1, 5, 6].

Although researchers have tried to probe the heritability of anxiety with studies of twin pairs, first-degree relatives, or big samples of anxiety-diagnosed patients,

IntechOpen

findings are inconsistent and could not be replicated [7–9], so there is no clear evidence to suggest a genetic component in the development of anxiety.

The assessment and treatment of childhood disorders are challenging because this population should not be compared to adults. Children and adolescent have their own features (e.g., difficulty to concentrate in school tasks, decreased academic or athletic performance, avoidance, "clinging" behavior, and tantrum [10]) which are in complex interaction with social and physiological environment.

In the similar way in young rats, anxiety has particular characteristics, and manifestation differs with age, e.g., in the elevated plus maze, young rodents (males and females) have high anxiety levels that increase with age [11]. However, adolescent females with food deprivation have lower anxiety level compared to adult rats [12]; these findings suggest that infantile and juvenile stages constitute a period of transition toward adulthood.

Therefore, the objective of this chapter is to review preclinical findings of experimental anxiety with pharmacological manipulations in young rats. This chapter will provide data from preclinical studies which are encouraged to a better comprehension of anxiety before adulthood.

2. Neurobiology of anxiety

Anxiety is a disorder of complex etiology, which includes stressful, environmental, epigenetic, social, and psychological factors that modify neurotransmission systems such as serotonergic, noradrenergic, dopaminergic, and glutamatergic [13–16]. The most studied neurobiological mechanism is the monoaminergic hypothesis, since clinically effective anxiolytic drugs have their place of action on various monoamines, such as serotonin (5-HT), noradrenaline (NE), and dopamine (DA), neurotransmitters involved in the pathogenesis of anxiety [13, 17]. However, in recent years attention has focused on alterations of the hypothalamic-pituitary-adrenal axis (HPA), neuroplasticity, neurogenesis, and inflammatory response [18], opening a new paradigm for the study of the biological bases of anxiety.

The amygdala is the main brain region involved in the processing of fear information by integrating prior learning and incoming sensory information from cortical and subcortical regions [19]. In anxiety disorders it is common to observe a decreased inhibitory neurotransmission mediated by gamma-aminobutyric acid (GABA), an increase in excitatory neurotransmission mediated by glutamate [20], as well as the interruption of fight-or-flight response mechanism regulated by the HPA axis with participation of emotional processing structures including the amygdala, hypothalamus, periaqueductal gray substance, and hippocampus and chemical mediators such as corticotropin-releasing factor, glutamate, and neuropeptides (substance P, neuropeptide Y, oxytocin, orexin, and galanin) [18, 20].

Unpredictable chronic mild stress increases glutamatergic neurotransmission and decreases prefrontal cortex (PFC) function in rats which display anxiety-like behavior [20], and the imbalance between neuronal excitation and inhibition in the medial prefrontal cortex, hippocampus, and amygdala contributes to the development of emotional disorders such as anxiety [21]. Chronic dexamethasone produces deficient learning and decreased pyramidal neurons in CA3 of the hippocampus in rats [22]. These findings lead to improper process of the cognitive responses to face aversive situations.

Glucocorticoids like corticosterone in rats can also alter the functional brain connections responsible for the emotional processing; for example, chronic stress decreases cognitive function due to loss of projections from the basolateral amygdala to the medial prefrontal cortex [23]. These data together indicate that if the organism remains in a state that deteriorates its homeostasis with alterations in the functionality of the HPA axis, responsible for regulating the response to stress, it leads to the development of diseases such as anxiety [21]. Thus, the secretion of hormones, such as glucocorticoids, catecholamines, growth hormone, and prolactin, promotes adaptive responses, but physiopathological processes are triggered when the response is excessive [24, 25].

On the other hand, glutamate is an excitatory neurotransmitter that acts through different types of N-methyl-D-aspartate (NMDA) and non-NMDA receptors. This neurotransmitter has been associated with anxiety since the increase of brain glutamate/glutamine levels induced by monosodium glutamate produces anxiety-like behavior measured in two models of anxiety, the open field test and the elevated plus maze [26]. In consistency the antagonism of NMDA receptors promotes anxiolytic-like behavior in experimental animal models of open field and marble burying [16].

3. Anxiety animal models

Animal models help to understand the physiopathology of some human diseases, the development of new therapeutic options, as well as the evaluation of the existing ones to identify other relevant effects [27]. Additionally, animals are relatively easy to obtain, maintain, and manipulate. They have broad reproducibility and involve less investment compared with clinical studies.

Our interest is situated in animal models of mental disorders associated to altered emotions. In the book *The Expression of the Emotions in Man and Animals*, Darwin makes it clear that through behavioral patterns, animals have the capacity to express their emotions [28]. Based on this capacity, a wide range of animal models have been developed, which allow us to understand some aspects of various psychiatric disorders as anxiety. Although it is not possible to fully model the complexity of human psychopathology, the physiological, anatomical, and genetic similarities allow us to understand, with limitations, the neurobiological basis of human diseases, as anxiety.

Animal models are very useful approaches at preclinical research to study anxiety and the closest possible to the anxiety disorders described in the DSM-5 which could occur at childhood and adolescence and not only in adults. **Table 1** shows some human anxiety disorders that can be studied in laboratory rats.

The animal models mentioned in **Table 1** are used to study anxiety disorders and the effectiveness of several pharmacological treatments. These models evaluate conditioned or unconditioned responses to novel or stressful stimuli, measuring

Human condition	Rodent model	Reference
Generalized anxiety, posttraumatic stress	Elevated plus maze, defensive burying test, marble burying, open field test, T-maze	[29–33]
Specific phobia: Photophobia, Social phobia, Agoraphobia	Light–dark box, social interaction test, hole board	[33]
Separation anxiety disorder	Maternal separation	[34]
Panic disorder	T-maze	[31–33]
Selective mutism	Social interaction test (with measure of pup ultrasound vocalizations during the test)	[35, 36]

Table 1.
Anxiety disorders and their experimental model used at young age.

Kind of validity	Aspect of validity	Object of validity (animal/human similarity of...)
Homological validity	Species validity	Species
	Strain validity	Strain
Pathogenic validity	Ontopathogenic validity	Interaction transforming an initial organism into a vulnerable organism
	Triggering validity	Interaction transforming an initial or a vulnerable organism into a pathological organism
Mechanistic validity		Theoretical cognitive or neurobiological mechanisms producing the observable effects of the disease
Face validity	Ethological validity	Behavioral symptoms of the disease
	Biomarker validity	Biomarkers associated with the disease
Predictive validity	Induction validity	Relation between the triggering factor and the observable effects of the disease
	Remission validity	Relation between the therapeutic agent and the observable effects of the disease

Source: Belzung and Lemoine [40].

Table 2.
Update of validity criteria for animal models.

behavioral or physiological responses in accordance to international laws that regulate the use of laboratory animals, with the aim of minimizing their use, pain, and stress [37].

Animal models are accepted as useful tools for studying human pathologies if they meet the criteria proposed by Willner [38] which include (i) predictive validity consisting of the similarity in the production of alterations of the human pathological state with the model and based on the sensitivity and specificity of the drugs used to reverse them; (ii) nominal or appearance validity, consisting of the similarity between the phenomena observed in the modeled and the human disorder; and (iii) construct validity which is the evaluation of the theoretical state in the condition under study, which should resemble the theoretical symptomatology of the human disorder in the animal model used for its study [38, 39]. These criteria continue evolving to have a more relevant approach to the human condition; **Table 2** summarizes the proposal of Belzung and Lemoine [40] that reformulates the classical criteria.

The young age for the purpose of this chapter means the first period of life, from 0 to 8 weeks in rats, since offspring depends from the dams to get nutrition and physical, intellectual, and social growth. While in humans there are already six age stages of development (neonatal, infant, childhood, juvenile, adulthood, and elderly), similarly the same can be identified in laboratory rats to research clinical conditions at preclinical level. In consistency with the validity criteria to study anxiety in childhood and adolescence at preclinical level, researchers should employ animal subjects at similar stages of development that can be observed in **Table 3**.

Behavioral and physiological responses activated by stress are similar in animals and humans. Thus, stress as a predisposing factor of anxiety can be experienced in several forms and produce nonadaptative responses depending on duration and intensity in animals. It is well-known that adverse experiences during sensitive developmental periods such as childhood and adolescence increase the predisposition to the development of neuropsychiatric disorders at the same age and later in adulthood [44]. In this sense, the preclinical study of anxiety involves experimental

Human age	Rat age	Development stage
0–24 months	0–28 days	Neonatal, lactating, infant
2–11 years	—	Childhood
12–18 years	29–55 days	Peripuberal, juvenile, adolescent
19–64 years	56 days–10 months	Adulthood
65 years	11 months	Older adult, elderly, aged

Table 3.
Comparison of the developmental stages between human and rat [41–43].

manipulations that generate stress responses during human childhood- and adolescence-like ages and allow us to observe some features of the disorders.

Some stressors used in infant and juvenile rats are chronic and unpredictable mild stress, space restriction, forced swimming, and maternal separation, among others. For example, 60 min of space restriction stress in rats at 30, 45, and 60 postnatal days (PND) increases plasma corticosterone levels and c-Fos protein expression in the amygdala and brain stem, suggesting a greater predisposition to the development of anxiety disorders [45]. Social stress in juvenile rats produces anorexic-like behavior in female mice [46].

Rats of 28 PND display behavioral responses suggestive of anxiety in defensive burying test (increase in burying time), an effect that is reversed by the administration of 1 mg/kg diazepam [30]. Stress by swimming produces a state of anxiety in 21 PND rats evaluated in the elevated plus maze (lower time spent in open arms and higher anxiety index) which is reversed by half of the adult effective dose (0.5 mg/kg diazepam), further suggesting that the infant rats are seemingly more sensitive to low dose of diazepam than adult rats, which is relevant for clinical applications [29].

The underlying mechanisms of anxiety disorders associated with the disruption of the mother-child relations at early stages are still unknown, but animal models of maternal separation can help to reproduce the molecular changes at the central nervous system responsible for anxiety-like behavior. For example, maternal separation in rodents has been shown to induce hyperactivity of the HPA increasing plasma corticosterone concentrations [47], where maternal deprivation for 15 and 180 min from 2 to 14 PND alters the mRNA mineralocorticoid and glucocorticoid receptors in the dentate gyrus of the hippocampus which is accompanied by hypersecretion of adrenocorticotropic hormone and corticosterone in plasma [48]. This is important because at least in animal models, an increase in plasma corticosterone concentrations is related to anxiety-like behaviors [49–51].

Thus, dysregulation of the HPA axis may be a marker of vulnerability to anxiety [48], where the HPA axis may be affected by the postnatal adversity induced by maternal separation [52]. Furthermore, 4–8 h maternal separation from 2 to 21 PND in male C57BL/6 mice increases anxiety-like behaviors in social preference test and in the elevated plus maze (reduction of time spent into open arms), which was related to an increase in IL-1β in the hippocampus, PFC, and serum [53]. Therefore, the inflammatory process induced by maternal separation affects two brain structures related to the pathophysiology of anxiety, i.e., the hippocampus and prefrontal cortex [53].

Maternal deprivation can also affect the brain development of rats, because 24 h of maternal deprivation increases the rate of cell death by labeling the 3′ end of DNA fragments using terminal transferase in the cerebral cortex and hippocampus in 12 PND rats, in addition to an increase in apoptosis-related proteins such as Bax and Blc-x in the frontal cortex. However, at 20 PND cell death is not as marked as in PND 12; therefore, maternal deprivation exerts a greater effect on immature neurons which are more vulnerable [47].

Similarly, in male Sprague Dawley rat pups, maternal separation from 2 to 21 PND for 3 h each day affects the serotonergic system, decreasing the number of positive cells to the expression of tryptophan hydroxylase (TPH) and 5-HT, identified with immunohistochemistry in the dorsal raphe nucleus, in addition to increasing pro-apoptotic proteins (cytochrome c, Bax, and caspase-3) and reactive oxygen species (H_2O_2) in the same brain nucleus, where these changes were again related to an increase in anxiety-like behaviors in the elevated plus maze and the open field test [54].

It should be noted that the dorsal raphe nucleus is a structure that participates in stress processes and mood disorders [55] and the induction of adverse effects in early life could indirectly generate a malfunction of the dorsal raphe nucleus and the serotonergic system which in the long term induces anxiety-like behaviors. Thus, maternal deprivation during critical periods of development will alter the functioning and brain wiring of infants exerting a risk factor for psychiatric disorders.

Social isolation is another factor of adversity in early stage of development that has been studied in basic research. Six hours of social isolation each day from 21 to 30 PND or from 21 to 40 PND in Wistar Kyoto rats reduced time and open arm entries and increased anxiety index in the elevated plus maze with respect to the subjects that remained in a group [56]. These findings could be related to a reduction of neurotrophic factors (BDNF, NGF, Arc), neurogenesis markers (Ki-67, BrdU), and the loss of density of dendritic spines in the hippocampus of the rat exposed to social isolation from 21 to 49 PND which can be reversed after the resocialization of experimental subjects [57]. The above shows how social isolation can affect neurotrophic processes and therefore impact the neuronal plasticity of the hippocampus, which could be indirectly generating negative effects on mood.

4. Experimental pharmacology of anxiety

Anxiety disorders in children and adolescents include symptoms which are similar to adults such as headache, fatigue, muscle tension, shortness of breath, and gastrointestinal problems, among others, as well as typical manifestations of the scholar child such as difficulty to concentrate in school tasks and decreased academic or athletic performance, accompanied by fear, avoidance, "clinging" behavior, and tantrum [10].

Research about the treatment of anxiety disorders during the first 18 years of life continues growing. The pharmacological approach to reverse anxiety disorders includes the selective serotonin reuptake inhibitors (SSRIs) like fluoxetine, fluvoxamine, and sertraline and serotonin norepinephrine reuptake inhibitors (SNRIs) like duloxetine as first-line treatment [58, 59], tricyclic antidepressants like clomipramine as second option [58], alpha-2A-adrenergic receptor agonist like guanfacine [60, 61], and benzodiazepines like diazepam as alternative treatment lines [62], drugs that have been evaluated with the support of animal models. **Table 4** resumes the results of some studies that evaluate the anxiolytic potential of substances evaluated using animal models of experimental anxiety at young age submitted to some stressors.

Interesting findings show that the pharmacological approaches in infant and adolescent rats are different from those of adults. The result is that specific adjustments should be applied if hypothesis are made to prove in young rats. Finally, all the attempts to increase the literature of anxiety in young subjects are useful

Stressor	Result	Drug	Reference
Ethanol acute administration at 7–30 PND	Open field test: hyperlocomotion at 14 PND and reduced time spent in the center of the open field, suggesting a state of anxiety, both effects reversed with omega 3	Omega-3 (720 mg/kg)	[63]
Maternal separation at 0–27 PND	Elevated plus maze: probiotic treatment increased time spent in open arms Light–dark box: probiotics reduced latency to lighted compartment	*Lactobacillus rhamnosus* strain R0011 (95%) and *Lactobacillus helveticus* R0052 (5%)	[64]
Single stress session of forced swim for 15 min at 21 PND	Elevated plus maze: stress reduced open arm time spent and increased anxiety index, reversed with diazepam	Diazepam (0.5 mg/kg)	[29]
Open spaces and height; low-intensity electric shock at 28 PND	Elevated plus maze: A fatty acid mixture (FAM) increased time, entries, and percentage in open arms and reduced the anxiety index similar to diazepam Defensive burying test: FAM reduced burying time	Diazepam 1 mg/kg; FAM 1 ml/rat	[65]
Open spaces and height at 28 PND	Elevated plus maze: diazepam but no oleic acid increased time spent on open arms and reduced the anxiety index	Oleic acid (10, 20, 40, 60, and 80 μg/rat) Diazepam (1 mg/kg)	[66]
Low-intensity electric shock at 21 PND	Defensive burying test: diazepam produced the anxiolytic effect only in a modified smaller round device	Diazepam (1 mg/kg)	[30]

Table 4.
Effects of anxiolytic drugs evaluated in young animal subjected to behavioral test.

to extend the comprehension of this clinical condition in order to dedicate higher attention to stress factors associated with it.

5. Discussion

Anxiety disorders can appear from early life stages and have its own characteristics, so diagnosis and treatment require the same particularity. Despite this, the scientific literature on anxiety disorders at young stages of life is less abundant than studies in adults. Infant and juvenile population is heterogeneous and complex, so the experimental characteristics under which the studies are developed are determinants for the results obtained. Naturally, young experimental subjects show anxiety levels that could increase with age, regardless of gender [11]. Some examples of the lower anxiety observed in young rats compared to adults are observed in adolescent animals with food deprivation which display lower levels of anxiety than adults evaluated in the elevated plus maze [12]. Juvenile male and female rats coming from pregnant dams exposed to unescapable low-intensity foot electric shocks remained more time in the open arms and in the elevated plus maze compared to their adult age [67], while adolescent rats exposed to maternal separation have higher levels of exploration in a novel environment and lower levels of corticosterone after exposure to that environment, showing lower levels of anxiety, while these effects are not observed in rats evaluated in the adult stage [68].

Regarding the response to pharmacological treatments, our group reported that the minimum anxiolytic effective dose of diazepam for animals of 21 PND is 0.5 mg/kg, being half of the minimum effective dose for adults [29]. While the use of selective serotonin reuptake inhibitors (SSRIs) like fluoxetine (first-line treatment in clinical practice [62]) shows diverse results, ranging from the absence of anxiolytic effects of fluoxetine with acute and chronic treatment [69] until paradoxical anxiogenic effects [70], possible explanation for diverse unexpected fluoxetine effects on infant and juvenile anxiety is based on mechanism of action of fluoxetine and the treatment duration. At first, on acute treatment fluoxetine increases extracellular serotonin levels for inhibition of reuptake, and the neurotransmitter remains free to stimulate postsynaptic receptors explaining the transitory increase in anxiety levels when fluoxetine treatment begins [71]. Later with chronic fluoxetine, high concentrations of serotonin inhibit serotonergic neurons in the dorsal raphe nucleus, reducing serotonin production and anxiety [71].

Some limitations that researchers face are the differences in experimental conditions, age, and even strains, which can explain the variability of the results obtained by diverse research groups. Of course the transition of preclinical findings to human condition should be modest and responsible, so generalizations should be avoided. With this brief review, it is clear that the expression of anxiety depends on age and represents a challenge but also an opportunity to generate knowledge that increases the scope of preclinical research. The advantages to study preclinical anxiety may consist in the opportunity to know the neurobiology of the developing brain under stress and pharmacological conditions. These manipulations on an organ with a great plasticity at early stages would lead to better results with potential reversible effects before reaching adulthood. Future studies must be encouraged to extend literature of infant and juvenile anxiety from preclinical to clinical approach, which could prevent adult high incidence of this clinical and disabling condition.

6. Conclusion

Based on preclinical findings, stressors produce human-like alterations before adulthood. The consequences are brain changes that impact behavioral performance generating anxiety. These effects are studied in the field of the experimental anxiety to probe pharmacological substances in order to extend knowledge of mechanism of action of new molecules or their combination with other drugs. This chapter described some aspects of brain function during early postnatal development which involves a critical period of vulnerability to psychiatric conditions. Child and adolescent anxiety preclinical research must be extended in order to improve the knowledge of this clinical condition.

Acknowledgements

This chapter was partially supported by Cátedras CONACYT Grant #1840 (National Council for Science and Technology) to Gabriel Guillén-Ruiz. Ana Karen Limón-Vázquez and Margarita Hernández-Mixteco received fellowships from CONACYT (Reg: 480040 and 452396, respectively).

Conflict of interest

The authors declare no conflict of interest.

Author details

Gabriel Guillén-Ruiz[1]*, Blandina Bernal-Morales[2], César Soria-Fregozo[3], Emma Virginia Herrera-Huerta[4], Ana Karen Limón-Vázquez[5], Margarita Hernández-Mixteco[5] and Abraham Puga-Olguín[5]

1 Laboratory of Neurofarmacology, Cátedras CONACYT, Institute of Neuroetology, Universidad Veracruzana, Xalapa, Veracruz, Mexico

2 Laboratory of Neurofarmacology, Institute of Neuroetology, Universidad Veracruzana, Xalapa, Veracruz, Mexico

3 Laboratory of Biomedical Sciences/Histology, University Center of Los Lagos, University of Guadalajara, Lagos de Moreno, Jalisco, Mexico

4 Faculty of Chemical Sciences, Universidad Veracruzana, Orizaba, Veracruz, Mexico

5 Postgraduate Studies in Neuroethology. Institute of Neuroethology, Universidad Veracruzana, Xalapa, Veracruz, Mexico

*Address all correspondence to: gguillen@uv.mx

References

[1] Coles J, Lee A, Taft A, Mazza D, Loxton D. Childhood sexual abuse and its association with adult physical and mental health: Results from a national cohort of young Australian women. Journal of Interpersonal Violence. 2015;**30**(11):1929-1944. DOI: 10.1177/0886260514555270

[2] Simonds LM, Pons RA, Stone NJ, Warren F, John M. Adolescents with anxiety and depression: Is social recovery relevant? Clinical Psychology and Psychotherapy. 2014;**21**(4):289-298. DOI: 10.1002/cpp.1841

[3] Battaglia M, Bertella S, Politi E, Bernardeschi L, Perna G, Gabriele A, et al. Age at onset of panic disorder: Influence of familial liability to the disease and of childhood separation anxiety disorder. The American Journal of Psychiatry. 1995;**152**(9):1362-1364. DOI: 10.1176/ajp.152.9.1362

[4] Dhakal S, Niraula S, Sharma NP, Sthapit S, Bennett E, Vaswani A, et al. History of abuse and neglect and their associations with mental health in rescued child labourers in Nepal. The Australian and New Zealand Journal of Psychiatry. 2019:4867419853882. DOI: 10.1177/0004867419853882

[5] Berzenski SR, Yates TM. Classes and consequences of multiple maltreatment: A person-centered analysis. Child Maltreatment. 2011;**16**(4):250-261. DOI: 10.1177/1077559511428353

[6] Moore SE, Scott JG, Ferrari AJ, Mills R, Dunne MP, Erskine HE, et al. Burden attributable to child maltreatment in Australia. Child Abuse & Neglect. 2015;**48**:208-220. DOI: 10.1016/j.chiabu.2015.05.006

[7] Stein MB, Gelernter J. Genetic factors in social anxiety disorder. In: Weeks JW, editor. The Wiley Handbook of Social Anxiety Disorder. Chichester: John Wiley & Sons; 2014

[8] Shimada-Sugimoto M, Otowa T, Hettema JM. Genetics of anxiety disorders: Genetic epidemiological and molecular studies in humans. Psychiatry & Clinical Neurosciences. 2015;**69**(7):388-401. DOI: 10.1111/pcn.12291

[9] Dunn EC, Sofer T, Gallo LC, Gogarten SM, Kerr KF, Chen CY, et al. Genome-wide association study of generalized anxiety symptoms in the hispanic community health study/study of latinos. American Journal of Medical Genetics. Part B, Neuropsychiatric Genetics. 2017;**174**(2):132-143. DOI: 10.1002/ajmg.b.32448

[10] American Psychiatric Association. Diagnostic and Statistical Manual of Mental Disorders. 5th ed. Arlington, VA: American Psychiatric Association; 2013

[11] Lynn DA, Brown GR. The ontogeny of anxiety-like behavior in rats from adolescence to adulthood. Developmental Psychobiology. 2010;**52**(8):731-739. DOI: 10.1002/dev.20468

[12] Genn RF, Tucci SA, Thomas A, Edwards JE, File SE. Age associated sex differences in response to food deprivation in two animal tests of anxiety. Neuroscience & Biobehavioral Reviews. 2003;**27**:155-161. DOI: 10.1016/s0149-7634(03)00017-4

[13] Keck ME, Sartori SB, Welt T, Müller MB, Ohl F, Holsboer F, et al. Differences in serotonergic neurotransmission between rats displaying high or low anxiety/depression-like behaviour: Effects of chronic paroxetine treatment. Journal of Neurochemistry. 2005;**92**(5):1170-1179. DOI: 10.1111/j.1471-4159.2004.02953.x

[14] Borodovitsyna O, Flamini MD, Chandler DJ. Acute stress persistently alters locus coeruleus function and anxiety-like behavior in adolescent rats. Neuroscience. 2018;**373**:7-19. DOI: 10.1016/j.neuroscience.2018.01.020

[15] Malikowska-Racia N, Salat K, Nowaczyk A, Fijalkowski L, Popik P. Dopamine D2/D3 receptor agonists attenuate PTSD-like symptoms in mice exposed to single prolonged stress. Neuropharmacology. 2019;**155**:1-9. DOI: 10.1016/j.neuropharm.2019.05.012

[16] Zhan Y, Xia J, Wang X. Effects of glutamate-related drugs on anxiety and compulsive behavior in rats with obsessive-compulsive disorder. International Journal of Neuroscience. 2019:1-13. DOI: 10.1080/00207454.2019.1684276

[17] McElligott ZA, Fox ME, Walsh PL, Urban DJ, Ferrel MS, Roth BL, et al. Noradrenergic synaptic function in the bed nucleus of the stria terminalis varies in animal models of anxiety and addiction. Neuropsychopharmacology. 2013;**38**(9):1665-1673. DOI: 10.1038/npp.2013.63

[18] Haj-Mirzaian A, Amiri S, Kordjazy N, Momeny M, Razmi A, Rahimi-Balaei M, et al. Lithium attenuated the depressant and anxiogenic effect of juvenile social stress through mitigating the negative impact of interlukin-1β and nitric oxide on hypothalamic-pituitary-adrenal axis function. Neuroscience. 2016;**315**:271-285. DOI: 10.1016/j.neuroscience.2015.12.024

[19] Selleck RA, Zhang W, Samberg HD, Padival M, Rosenkranz JA. Limited prefrontal cortical regulation over the basolateral amygdala in adolescent rats. Scientific Reports. 2018;**8**(1):17171. DOI: 10.1038/s41598-018-35649-0

[20] Shepard R, Coutellier L. Changes in the prefrontal glutamatergic and parvalbumin systems of mice exposed to unpredictable chronic stress. Molecular Neurobiology. 2018;**55**(3):2591-2602. DOI: 10.1007/s12035-017-0528-0

[21] Lovelock DF, Deak T. Acute stress imposed during adolescence yields heightened anxiety in Sprague Dawley rats that persists into adulthood: Sex differences and potential involvement of the medial amygdala. Brain Research. 2019;**1723**:146392. DOI: 10.1016/j.brainres.2019.146392

[22] Cerqueira JJ, Pêgo JM, Taipa R, Bessa JM, Almeida OF, Sousa N. Morphological correlates of corticosteroid-induced changes in prefrontal cortex-dependent behaviors. The Journal of Neuroscience. 2005;**25**:7792-7800. DOI: 10.1523/JNEUROSCI.1598-05.2005

[23] Duvarci S, Paré D. Glucocorticoids enhance the excitability of principal basolateral amygdala neurons. The Journal of Neuroscience. 2007;**27**:4482-4491. DOI: 10.1523/JNEUROSCI.0680-07.2007

[24] Telegdy G, Schally AV. Neurotransmitter-mediated action of an antagonist of growth hormone-releasing hormone on anxiolysis in mice. Behavioural Brain Research. 2012;**233**(1):232-236. DOI: 10.1016/j.bbr.2012.04.011

[25] Zamorano M, Ledesma-Colunga MG, Adán N, Vera-Massieu C, Lemini M, Méndez I, et al. Prolactin-derived vasoinhibins increase anxiety- and depression-related behaviors. Psychoneuroendocrinology. 2014;**44**:123-132. DOI: 10.1016/j.psyneuen.2014.03.006

[26] Onaolapo OJ, Aremu OS, Onaolapo AY. Monosodium glutamate-associated alterations in open field, anxiety-related and conditioned place preference behaviours in mice.

Naunyn-Schmiedeberg's Archives of Pharmacology. 2017;**390**(7):677-689. DOI: 10.1007/s00210-017-1371-6

[27] Valdés SM, Álvarez AL, Del Barrio G. Los modelos animales en la evaluación preclínica de antivirales contra los virus del herpes simple [Animal models in preclinical evaluation of antiviral against herpes virus]. Revista de Salud Animal. 2009;**31**(2):86-92

[28] Darwin C. The Expression of the Emotions in Man and Animals. London: John Murray; 1872

[29] Bernal-Morales B, Guillén-Ruiz G, Cueto-Escobedo J, Rodríguez-Landa JF, Contreras CM. Sensitivity to diazepam after a single session of forced swim stress in weaning Wistar rats. Acta Pharmaceutica (Zagreb, Croatia). 2018;**68**(3):381-388. DOI: 10.2478/acph-2018-0027

[30] Cueto-Escobedo J, Contreras CM, Bernal-Morales B, Guillén-Ruiz G, Rodríguez-Landa JF. Defensive burying test in postweaning rats: Use of a small round chamber. Behavioural Pharmacology. 2013;**24**(8):693-698. DOI: 10.1097/FBP.0000000000000008

[31] Baker S, Chebli M, Rees S, Lemarec N, Godbout R, Bielajew C. Effects of gestational stress: 1. Evaluation of maternal and juvenile offspring behavior. Brain Research. 2008;**1213**:98-110. DOI: 10.1016/j.brainres.2008.03.035

[32] Campos AC, Fogaça MV, Aguiar DC, Guimarães FS. Animal models of anxiety disorders and stress. Brazilian Journal of Psychiatry. 2013;**35**(2):S101-S111. DOI: 10.1590/1516-4446-2013-1139

[33] Balemans MC, Huibers MM, Eikelenboom NW, Kuipers AJ, van Summeren RC, Pijpers MM, et al. Reduced exploration, increased anxiety, and altered social behavior: Autistic-like features of euchromatin histone methyltransferase 1 heterozygous knockout mice. Behavioural Brain Research. 2010;**208**(1):47-55. DOI: 10.1016/j.bbr.2009.11.008

[34] Isobe A, Kawaguchi M. Relationship between motor function and ultrasonic vocalizations induced by maternal separation in rat pups. The Journal of Veterinary Medical Science. 2019;**81**(2):287-293. DOI: 10.1292/jvms.18-0604

[35] Al-Afif S, Staden M, Krauss JK, Schwabe K, Hermann EJ. Splitting of the cerebellar vermis in juvenile rats-effects on social behavior, vocalization and motor activity. Behavioural Brain Research. 2013;**250**:293-298. DOI: 10.1016/j.bbr.2013.05.013

[36] Al-Afif S, Krauss JK, Helms F, Angelov S, John N, Schwabe K, et al. Long-term impairment of social behavior, vocalizations and motor activity induced by bilateral lesions of the fastigial nucleus in juvenile rats. Brain Structure & Function. 2019;**224**(5):1739-1751. DOI: 10.1007/s00429-019-01871-3

[37] Hernández S. El modelo animal en las investigaciones biomédicas. Biomedicina. 2006;**2**(3):252-256

[38] Willner P. Methods for assessing the validity of animal models of human psychopathology. In: Boulton A et al., editors. Animal Models in Psychiatry I. USA: Humana Press; 1991

[39] Morrice JR, Gregory-Evans CY, Shaw CA. Animal models of amyotrophic lateral sclerosis: A comparison of model validity. Neural Regeneration Research. 2018;**13**(12):2050-2054. DOI: 10.4103/1673-5374.241445

[40] Belzung C, Lemoine M. Criteria of validity for animal models of psychiatric disorders: Focus on anxiety disorders

and depression. Biology of Mood & Anxiety Disorders. 2011;**1**(1):9. DOI: 10.1186/2045-5380-1-9

[41] Becú-Villalobos D, Lacau-Menguido IM. Control hormonal del desarrollo puberal en la rata hembra. Acta Physiologica et Pharmacologica Latino americana. 1990;**40**(1):1-17

[42] Spear LP. The adolescent brain and age-related manifestations. Neuroscience & Biobehavioral Reviews. 2000;**24**:417-463. DOI: 10.1016/s0149-7634(00)00014-2

[43] World Health Organization. e-Library of Evidence for Nutrition Actions (eLENA): life course [Internet]. 2019. Available from: https://www.who.int/elena/life_course/en/ [Accessed: 13 November 2019]

[44] Lenze SN, Xiong C, Sheline YI. Childhood adversity predicts earlier onset of major depression but not reduced hippocampal volume. Psychiatry Research. 2008;**162**(1):39-49. DOI: 10.1016/j.pscychresns.2007.04.004

[45] Kovács LÁ, Schiessl JA, Nafz AE, Csernus V, Gaszner B. Both basal and acute restraint stress-induced c-Fos expression is influenced by age in the extended amygdala and brainstem stress centers in male rats. Frontiers in Aging Neuroscience. 2018;**10**:248. DOI: 10.3389/fnagi.2018.00248

[46] Madra M, Zeltser LM. BDNF-Val66Met variant and adolescent stress interact to promote susceptibility to anorexic behavior in mice. Translational Psychiatry. 2016;**6**:e776. DOI: 10.1038/tp.2016.35

[47] Zhang LX, Levine S, Dent G, Zhan Y, Xing G, Okimoto D, et al. Maternal deprivation increases cell death in the infant rat brain. Developmental Brain Research. 2002;**133**:1-11. DOI: 10.1016/s0926-6410(01)00118-5

[48] Ladd CO, Huot RL, Thrivikraman KV, Nemeroff CB, Plotsky PM. Long-term adaptations in glucocorticoid receptor and mineralocorticoid receptor mRNA and negative feedback on the hypothalamo-pituitary-adrenal axis following neonatal maternal separation. Biological Psychiatry. 2004;**55**(4):367-375. DOI: 10.1016/j.biopsych.2003.10.007

[49] Vega-Rivera NM, Fernández-Guasti A, Ramírez-Rodríguez G, Estrada-Camarena E. Acute stress further decreases the effect of ovariectomy on immobility behavior and hippocampal cell survival in rats. Psychoneuroendocrinology. 2013;**38**:1407-1417. DOI: 10.1016/j.psyneuen.2012.12.008

[50] Wang Z, Gu J, Wang X, Xie K, Luan Q, Wan N, et al. Antidepressant-like activity of resveratrol treatment in the forced swim test and tail suspension test in mice: The HPA axis, BDNF expression and phosphorylation of ERK. Pharmacology, Biochemistry & Behavior. 2013;**112**:104-110. DOI: 10.1016/j.pbb.2013.10.007

[51] Vega-Rivera NM, Fernández-Guasti A, Ramírez-Rodríguez G, Estrada-Camarena E. Forced swim and chronic variable stress reduced hippocampal cell survival in OVX female rats. Behavioural Brain Research. 2014;**270**:48-55. DOI: 10.1016/j.bbr.2014.05.033

[52] Houwing DJ, Ramsteijn AS, Riemersma IW, Olivier JDA. Maternal separation induces anhedonia in female heterozygous serotonin transporter knockout rats. Behavioural Brain Research. 2019;**356**:204-207. DOI: 10.1016/j.bbr.2018.08.031

[53] Wang Q, Dong X, Wang Y, Liu M, Sun A, Li N, et al. Adolescent escitalopram prevents the effects of maternal separation on depression- and anxiety-like behaviours and regulates

the levels of inflammatory cytokines in adult male mice. International Journal of Developmental Neuroscience. 2017;**62**:37-45. DOI: 10.1016/j.ijdevneu.2017.07.007

[54] Park SS, Park HS, Kim CJ, Baek SS, Kim TW. Exercise attenuates maternal separation-induced mood disorder-like behaviors by enhancing mitochondrial functions and neuroplasticity in the dorsal raphe. Behavioural Brain Research. 2019;**372**:112049. DOI: 10.1016/j.bbr.2019.112049

[55] Donner NC, Handa RJ. Estrogen receptor beta regulates the expression of tryptophanhydroxylase 2 mRNA within serotonergic neurons of the rat dorsal raphe nuclei. Neuroscience. 2009;**163**(2):705-718. DOI: 10.1016/j.neuroscience.2009.06.046

[56] Shetty RA, Sadananda M. Immediate and delayed anxiety- and depression-like profiles in the adolescent Wistar-Kyoto rat model of endogenous depression following postweaning social isolation. Behavioural Brain Research. 2017;**320**:323-332. DOI: 10.1016/j.bbr.2016.12.030

[57] Biggio F, Mostallino MC, Talani G, Locci V, Mostallino R, Calandra G, et al. Social enrichment reverses the isolation-induced deficits of neuronal plasticity in the hippocampus of male rats. Neuropharmacology. 2019;**151**:45-54. DOI: 10.1016/j.neuropharm.2019.03.030

[58] da Costa CZ, de Morais RM, Zanetta DM, Turkiewicz G, Lotufo Neto F, Morikawa M, et al. Comparison among clomipramine, fluoxetine, and placebo for the treatment of anxiety disorders in children and adolescents. Journal of Child & Adolescent Psychopharmacology. 2013;**23**(10):687-692. DOI: 10.1089/cap.2012.0110

[59] Locher C, Koechlin H, Zion SR, Werner C, Pine DS, Kirsch I, et al. Efficacy and safety of selective serotonin reuptake inhibitors, serotonin-norepinephrine reuptake inhibitors, and placebo for common psychiatric disorders among children and adolescents: A systematic review and meta-analysis. JAMA Psychiatry. 2017;**74**(10):1011-1020. DOI: 10.1001/jamapsychiatry.2017.2432

[60] Dobson ET, Bloch MH, Strawn JR. Efficacy and tolerability of pharmacotherapy for pediatric anxiety disorders: A network meta-analysis. Journal of Clinical Psychiatry. 2019;**80**(1). pii: 17r12064. DOI: 10.4088/JCP.17r12064

[61] Strawn JR, Compton SN, Robertson B, Albano AM, Hamdani M, Rynn MA. Extended release guanfacine in pediatric anxiety disorders: A pilot, randomized, placebo-controlled trial. Journal of Child & Adolescent Psychopharmacology. 2017;**27**(1):29-37. DOI: 10.1089/cap.2016.0132

[62] Rynn M, Puliafico A, Heleniak C, Rikhi P, Ghalib K, Vidair H. Advances in pharmacotherapy for pediatric anxiety disorders. Depression and Anxiety. 2011;**28**(1):76-87. DOI: 10.1002/da.20769

[63] Balaszczuk V, Salguero JA, Villarreal RN, Scaramuzza RG, Mendez S, Abate P. Hyperlocomotion and anxiety-like behavior induced by binge ethanol exposure in rat neonates. Possible ameliorative effects of omega 3. Behavioural Brain Research. 2019;**372**:112022. DOI: 10.1016/j.bbr.2019.112022

[64] Peng HH, Tsai TC, Huang WY, Wu HM, Hsu KS. Probiotic treatment restores normal developmental trajectories of fear memory retention in maternally separated infant rats. Neuropharmacology. 2019;**153**:53-62. DOI: 10.1016/j.neuropharm.2019.04.026

[65] Bernal-Morales B, Cueto-Escobedo J, Guillén-Ruiz G, Rodríguez-Landa JF, Contreras CM. A fatty acids mixture reduces anxiety-like

behaviors in infant rats mediated by $GABA_A$ receptors. BioMed Research International. 2017;**2017**:8798546. DOI: 10.1155/2017/8798546

[66] Guillén-Ruiz G, Bernal-Morales B, Contreras CM, Cueto-Escobedo J, Rodríguez-Landa JF. Oleic acid produces motor incoordination and hypoactivity in infant Wistar rats through $GABA_A$ receptors. Journal of Psychiatry & Neuroscience. 2016;**4**:18-25. DOI: 10.11648/j.ajpn.20160402.11

[67] Estanislau C, Morato S. Behavior ontogeny in the elevated plus-maze: Prenatal stress effects. International Journal of Developmental Neuroscience. 2006;**24**(4):255-262. DOI: 10.1016/j.ijdevneu.2006.03.001

[68] Yoo SB, Kim BT, Kim JY, Ryu V, Kang DW, Lee JH, et al. Adolescence fluoxetine increases serotonergic activity in the raphe-hippocampus axis and improves depression-like behaviors in female rats that experienced neonatal maternal separation. Psychoneuroendocrinology. 2013;**38**(6):777-788. DOI: 10.1016/j.psyneuen.2012.08.013

[69] Lapmanee S, Charoenphandhu J, Charoenphandhu N. Beneficial effects of fluoxetine, reboxetine, venlafaxine, and voluntary running exercise in stressed male rats with anxiety- and depression-like behaviors. Behavioural Brain Research. 2013;**250**:316-325. DOI: 10.1016/j.bbr.2013.05.018

[70] Handley SL, McBlane JW. Opposite effects of fluoxetine in two animal models of anxiety. British Journal of Pharmacology. 1992;**107**:446

[71] Farhan M, Haleem DJ. Anxiolytic profile of fluoxetine as monitored following repeated administration in animal rat model of chronic mild stress. Saudi Pharmaceutical Journal. 2016;**24**(5):571-578. DOI: 10.1016/j.jsps.2015.03.006

Chapter 7

Comprehensive Attention with a Harm Reduction Perspective for Psychoactive Substances Consumers in a Third Level Hospital

María Angélica Ocampo, César Guillermo Popoca, Abraham Sánchez, Catalina Casillas and Raúl Cicero

Abstract

The great problem of addictions during the last five decades has been investigated through the behavioral analysis of social determinants involving multiple risk factors of initiation and maintenance of legal and illegal substances consumption, as well as the search of protective factors that allow preventing and achieving abstinence of drug abuse. Currently there is no solution and we are at the crossroads of lacking comprehensive attention, since there are treatments focused only on achieving abstinence and do not pay attention to the physical consequences of substance consumption, such as: infectious and non-communicable diseases. It is important to treat the addictions problem with a holistic approach, which facilitates access to effective medical services, based on scientific evidence, applied to adherence to treatment and adapted to patient diagnosis. With the aim of preventing or reducing the physical and mental damages that these substances can cause to the health of the users, allowing to achieve a better quality of life.

Keywords: addictions, behavior analysis, harm reduction, adherence to treatment, comprehensive attention

1. Introduction

Regarding *addictions* of psychoactive substances, there are multiple definitions since it is a multifactorial phenomenon ranging from the moment of the vital development in which the subject is, in which the gender influences the process of addition, both physically and socially, up to the pattern of consumption, the type of substance ingested, the route of administration, among others. However, one of the main characteristics of addiction is that it generates changes at a functional level in the brain by altering the reward and self-control systems [1]. According to the World Health Organization the addiction is a physical and psycho-emotional disease, related to a set of signs and symptoms, in which biological, genetic, psychological and social factors are compromised [2]. Considering that over the years new substances producing greater damage to consumers' health [3] have emerged, the WHO has made changes to the classification of substance abuse disorders, in order to improve the prevention and treatment of these problems, these modifications will be reflected in the CIE-11, which is expected to take effect in January 2022. So far, one of the effective models to follow in the intervention of addictions is the Harm Reduction to improve the quality of life of the substance abusers, with or without achieving abstinence, but improving physical and mental health [4].

2. Global epidemiology

Inequality at a global level represents a social problem that influenced the phenomenon of drug abuse, which has experienced a serious growth, since only in a decade the number of people abusing drugs increased by 30% worldwide, from 2009 with 210 million people to 2019 with 271 million consumers of psychoactive substances, representing 5.5% of the population between 15 and 64 years of age, of which 17 million abusers suffer from infectious diseases such as HIV/AIDS, Tuberculosis and Hepatitis C; in the latter, the main cause was the increase of "opioids" consumers, with approximately 53.4 million people consuming it worldwide, being the main responsible for the majority of the 585,000 deaths; in addition of the lost years of healthy life due to disabilities entitled to drug abuse, with about 42 million years of healthy life [5] (Cited [6]). Besides, an alarming fact are respiratory diseases, cardiovascular pathologies, as well as cancer associated with drug abuse, without undermining of deaths due to injected drugs overdose, with a higher risk of suicide, in addition to psychiatric comorbidities; being a focus of attention for health systems in the world since only 1 in 6 drug abusers receives medical treatment [7].

In America, the consumption of abused substances is not less alarming, considering that the start of the consumption of any psychoactive substance, including alcohol and tobacco, starts during high school and it is decreasing even further. An important fact in the continent is the systematic decrease shown by the use of tobacco over time, probably due to the creation of the WHO Framework Convention on Tobacco Control arising from the need to combat this pandemic in 2003 [8] and having a positive impact on the legislation of its use worldwide. In the America continent, tobacco shows decreases in its use in most of the countries monitoring it, as is the case in Chile, even with the highest level, going from 44 to 33.4% from 2000 to 2016 in the consumption of the last month; but in terms of alcohol consumption, there is a decrease in consumers but those that exist are taking more and more [9]; in the case of illegal drugs, trends in use are increasing, especially cannabis and cocaine. These increases in consumption have also been identified in other substances, such as new psychoactive substances (NPS), opioids and benzodiazepines, which produce new challenges for the treatment of patients with dependency, for public health and drug policies in general [10].

3. Epidemiology in Mexico

In Mexico, poppy cultivation had a 21% increase from 2016 to 2017, keeping the country in third place worldwide in its production [6], mainly in the "Golden Triangle" formed by Sonora, Durango and Chihuahua, north of Nayarit and the state of Guerrero, which responds to the socioeconomic situation of poverty in the population [7]. Our country has become the main distributor of the United States of America with 86% of the total of this drug [11].

According to the National Survey of Drug, Alcohol and Tobacco Consumption (ENCODAT) 2016–2017 [12], alcohol is the most consumed and 1.8 million people in the country already have dependence; while in the population from 12 to 65 years old, the excessive consumption of alcohol increased from 12.3% in 2011 to 19.8% in 2016.

Tobacco is the second most consumed psychoactive substance; its prevalence in the population from 12 to 65 years old remained stable between 2011 and 2016 with 17 and 17.6%, respectively [12].

The consumption of any illegal drug increased from 7.2% in 2011 to 9.9% in 2016, the preferred drugs abused at some time in life continue to be marijuana (8.6%) and cocaine (3.5%) [12]. The use of illicit drugs (marijuana, cocaine, heroin), substances of abuse (solvents and inhalants) and non-prescription drugs (stimulants, depressants), as well as new psychoactive substances, show a lower prevalence compared to tobacco and alcohol statistics. However, the seriousness of the matter is the severe damage they generate in the individual health, with implications for family members, the community and society in general, as it is associated with greater emphasis on insecurity and violence problems [13].

Regarding medical care, in the *Report on the situation of drug abuse in Mexico and its comprehensive care 2019*, from 2010 to 2017 of the 22,856 deaths directly related to drug abuse, the largest number with 21,920 are caused by the consumption of alcohol, this is the reason why it continues to be the main drug for which attention is requested in medical emergencies, followed by the consumption of cocaine, volatile solvents and marijuana. Among the diseases prior to admission due to medical emergency under the influence of a drug, the appearance of the following were mainly reported: musculoskeletal condition, alcoholic/substance psychosis, diabetes mellitus, gastritis, cirrhosis and hypertension. As relevant data in the last deaths register of 2017, in our country 2597 people died, of which the highest percentage of deaths were between 30 and 49 years of age [14] which are one of the most productive stages in the lives of human beings, reflecting the lack of effective educational activities and campaigns for the prevention and early and timely detection of conditions to guide consumers regarding these chronic degenerative non-communicable diseases (NCDs) that represent a serious problem for public health in Mexico. Only in 2016, two of the main health care institutions in our country, Instituto Mexicano del Seguro Social (IMSS) and Instituto de Servicio y Seguro Social de los Trabajadores del Estado (ISSSTE), together allocated 31.4% of their budget for the attention of diseases such as: diabetes, hypertension, renal impairment and cancer [15], being mainly those of greater demand, combined with the low budget that the Mexican health system has received and the lack of specialized coverage that prevents it from reaching poorer populations.

4. Psychosocial determinants of addictions and epigenetics

The coverage in universal health is a worldwide problem. The burden of a disease is observed in disadvantaged groups resulting in disability at a very young age. The dynamics in the social hierarchy and the social flow of the disease are the bases on which the Social Determinants of Health (SDH) model is based, explaining the majority of inequalities in and between countries when directing interventions in the structural determinants and intermediates underlying health inequity: the former includes the political and economic context where social hierarchical patterns originate, modify and maintain within cultural norms and values; these determinants shape the health of the individuals based on their social position, gender, age, employment, race and ethnic group, income, and education; while the intermediate determinants are the means by which the structural determinants operate, allowing the exposure to conditions damaging the health of the subject such as: housing quality, physical work environment, social support networks, healthy lifestyles, genetic factors, social cohesion and the structure of the health system [16, 17].

In Mexico, based on measurements carried out by the "Consejo Nacional de Evaluación de la Política de Desarrollo Social" (CONEVAL), some of the social determinants show that 52.4 million people are in poverty, which represents 41.9% in 2018 compared to 44.4% in 2008. On the other hand there are 9.3 million people in extreme poverty (7.4%) and 37.7 million vulnerable people due to social deprivations, whose main indicators of the total Mexican population include: educational lag (16.9%), access to health services (16.2%) access to social security (57.3%), access to food (20.4%), housing quality and spaces (11.1%) and access to basic housing services (19.8%) [18].

Therefore the social determinants describe addictions as a public health problem caused by the lack of a public health policy. The economic and basic education inequality, as structural determinants, hinder the development of all the physical and intellectual potential of people, since these would have to operate as protective factors in society; therefore, their absence affects and impacts directly on the intermediate determinants, which are distorted, when observed without a basic system in the health condition, in the family, culture and nutrition of the population to name the most important [19].

Consequently, addressing the risk factors fills the gaps that the traditional medical model has left in the search for the causes related to NCD and that will prevent its progress. The use of this concept has its importance and historical development in medicine with the improvement of techniques in the treatment of infectious diseases based on microbial theory, considering that humanity has gone through an epidemiological transition, in which the increase and appearing of non-communicable diseases, such as cardiovascular, cancer, chronic obstructive pulmonary disease and diabetes, cannot be treated as infectious diseases were treated, where there was a pathogen, because the causes of NCDs are multifactorial, among which the consumption of addictive substances, physical inactivity and deficit in eating behavior stand out [20].

Considering that the causal relationship with the health condition is different for each consumer, it will be difficult to identify a specific factor for each one. However, it has been possible to find functional relationships in which the consumption pattern will be characterized in the one hand by the type of substance abused, and in the other hand in the chain of functional background in the case of structural determinants, understood as "those circumstances in which people are born, grow, live, work and grow old as a result of the distribution of money, power and resources that will depend on the public policies adopted" [21] will play an important role.

Within each functional analysis of the behavior of drug abusers, they report in the background that the psychosocial determinants of addictions are in a cultural context that molds and shapes values in people, structuring their personality [22], which makes them more vulnerable to drug abuse in the short, medium or long term. The abuse of psychoactive substances operates as a positive reinforcement before situations that, after their consumption, are gratifying because allow avoiding such a displeasing situation for a moment [23], a feeling of relaxation due to excessive work hours, the attachment to consumers receiving support from the same when there is no affection in the family or the ease of consumption in recreational spaces such as bars, allows consumers to maintain unhealthy lifestyles [24].

The use of addictive substances is a complex behavior. To begin understanding the different variables related, it is necessary to comprehend that people are acquiring different behaviors based on learning, whether they are transmitted verbally, or if the person observes the behavior and then executes it [25].

As already mentioned, the etiology of the use of addictive substances is classified as multifactorial, because there is not only one factor determining an addictive behavior. But it can be confirmed that the main factors related to a substance abuse problem are usually environmental, psychological and genetic [7, 26]. Since the interaction between genes and the environment can cause the expression of genes to undergo some modification, i.e., the individual experience of consumers produces changes in genes, which in turn influence memory, cognition, emotions and behavior, it can lead to a psychiatric disorder [27]. Sometimes, these genetic changes are not reversible and, unfortunately, not only influence the person who uses addictive substances, but also can be inherited. Consequently, substance abuse decreases the quality of life of the current and future generations. Among the environmental factors that lead to epigenetic changes, the following stand out: prenatal and postnatal factors, such as malnutrition, drug abuse of the parents during pregnancy, abuse or stress [28]. To address the problem of substance abuse, the traditional medical model is insufficient to achieve adherence to treatment, because it only contemplates the biological factor. For that reason, it is relevant to focus the intervention towards a flexible treatment which adapts to the different factors influencing substance abuse. Interdisciplinary treatments have been reported to produce benefits to maintain or improve the quality of life of people with chronic degenerative diseases [29]. This style of treatment is characterized by relying on different areas of knowledge to improve or maintain effectively the health of people who consume addictive substances.

It is important to note that addictions treatment, although predominantly of a psychological type, must be duly complemented by medical specialists who focus their action not only on the pharmacological treatment of the addiction, while also emphasizing the timely diagnosis of conditions as well as the reference - counter-reference of patients with conditions, associated with consumption, as this action will be decisive in the adherence that drug abusers will have to the medical treatment and which, in turn, will promote their decision of abstinence [30] (**Figure 1**).

The definition based on the above, in which the strong relationship of the psychosocial determinants in addictions is observed, as well as some of the risk factors for medical and psychiatric comorbidities due to the use of addictive substances, becomes the implementation of treatments in the three levels of health care emergent; considering that entering in the topic of addictions is relatively new for health professionals, in addition to the fact that this interventions are not so simple, since treating an individual with addictions is carried out with marked parameters of preventive medicine and not only from the cure of the medical and psychiatric comorbidities that these consumptions cause. The treatment needs to be transdisciplinary and must include health protection, promotion and maintenance parameters, as well as the abstinence from substance abuse, since the user and abuse are committed in a multifactorial way.

Different treatments have been implemented in patients who have problems with the use of addictive substances. In the 60s, they were treated with psychological therapies with the aim of modifying behavior based on punishment. These patients have a high rate of remission that over time presented a relapse [31]. Interventions via telephone, online and self-help manuals are also effective but over the months the relapse rate was significant [32].

With the advance of research and the development of psychology, programs were created that tried to improve treatments to increase adherence to treatment. To be able to work with the problem of additions it was done from the multidisciplinary, involving different areas of knowledge in such a way that adequate

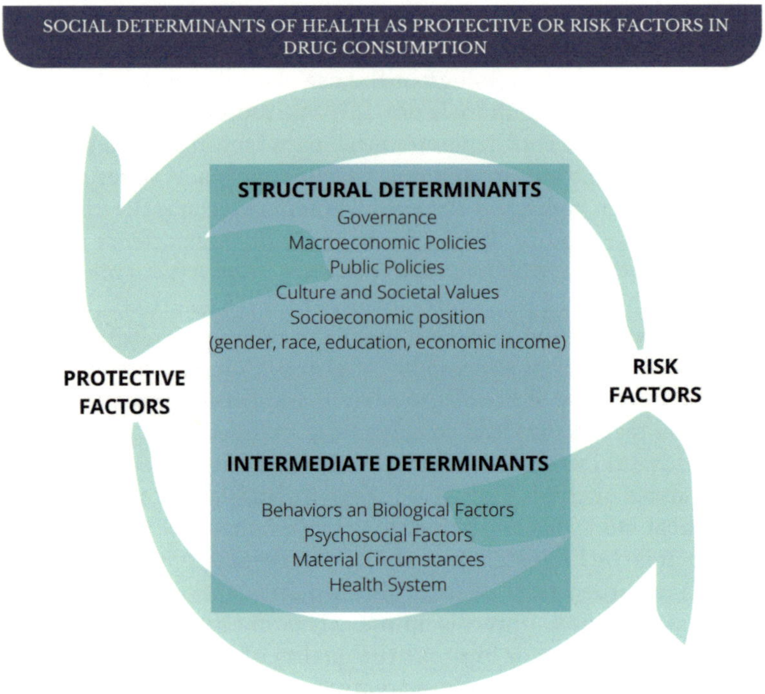

Figure 1.
Mexico presents inequality between its population and the social determinants allow us to understand the consumption of psychoactive substances in the country [18, 19].

treatments will be provided to maintain or improve the quality of life of patients. The results are positive and supported by different investigations.

A Meta-analysis conducted by Schwartz [33] to a total of 416 clinical trials of different treatments for smokers and complemented by Becoña [34] recognizes the relevance of multimodal or multidisciplinary treatments to achieve abstinence, placing them as the most effective treatment. These results are supported by the work of Sanz et al. [35] who provided interdisciplinary treatment for people who use tobacco, granted psychological treatment, supported by nicotine replacement therapies, bupropion and other medical alternatives according to the patient's characteristics. At the end of the treatment approximately 70% of the participants were in withdrawal.

It is suggested that integrated care may provide long-term benefits in terms of medical and wellness outcomes 6 months after treatment, for example Sterling [36] reports that in several studies conducted by Drug and Alcohol Research Team (DART) integrated care in the treatment of people with consumption of alcohol and other drugs and with medical or psychiatric conditions have 69% withdrawal compared to 55%. In a systematic review by Savic [37], it indicates that one of the objectives of comprehensive care is to improve the quality of life, incorporating the harm reduction strategy to achieve success. On the other hand, within the important strategies for comprehensive care, staff training, training on alcohol and other drugs to doctors who have no attention to consumers is relevant, the reference to other instances for medical care is also indicated as An important strategy.

5. Harm reduction

If we examine the increase in the use of legal and illegal psychoactive substances during the last five decades, they have led us to the search for the best clinical practices, in which their user will benefit from treatment and rehabilitation schemes to find the "cure"; that it is not only when consumption is abandoned in hospitalizations since, sadly for our health institutions, all the efforts made in these schemes do not contemplate the approaches for medical and psychiatric comorbidities derived from consumption, reducing the effectiveness from the discharge of the substance abusers, believing that the clinical setting that led them to this will not be repeated. Most of the time, when users are facing their daily life associated with consumption they restart the intake of psychoactive substances, discarding that all professional efforts in clinical treatments are extinguished with their relapse.

The World Drug Report [7] mentions the urgent need to redouble efforts in order to facilitate access to effective medical services, based on scientific evidence, in terms of prevention, treatment and care for people who consume psychoactive substances and desperately need them.

An example of these measures can be identified in the need to accelerate the accessibility to Hepatitis C treatment, a disease whose harmful health consequences for "drug" users are much greater than those of HIV/AIDS. It is very important to frame that in the latter, the transmission of the virus was one of the main diseases that emerged as an epidemic in the early 1980s through injected drugs (opiates) and at the end there will be the exchange of syringes in consumers of heroin in Liverpool or the decriminalization of the personal dose (amount without being lethal or illegal) in Holland in 1976 [38]. When total abstinence is not met, it is important to considered that one of the fundamental basis is to reduce or avoid further damage [39] by decreasing morbidity-mortality and achieving family stability and the possibility of obtaining and keeping a job, family, besides to health, which is a priority [40].

Mexico has also implemented projects for harm reduction, such as the Syringe Program, as well as Methadone substitution therapy in Ciudad Juárez and Tijuana, managed by Non Governmental Organizations [41], which support people with physiological dependencies to prevent them from sharing the same syringe and avoid more complications.

In the context of demonstrating the benefits that can be obtained through multidisciplinary treatments, in which the aim is to achieve comprehensive health and improve the quality of life of the patients who consume any substance harmful to their health, which leads to non-communicable and infectious diseases also by the relationship of unhealthy behaviors. *Harm Reduction* is one element where it has been proven that it is not only about abstinence of substance abuse, it is also reducing the risks and damages associated to it.

Due to the relevance of the application of this strategy, we will now discern its meaning and scope in the current medicine. *Reduction* comes from the Latin *reductio* and means "action of returning something where or how it was." Its lexical components are: the prefix re- (backwards); the word Damage (discomfort, pain, deterioration or injure) comes from the Latin *damnum* (condemnation, punishment) [42]. For purposes of having an understanding updated and focused on the objective of finding a definition expressing the subject under study regarding the chore of health professionals' work within the intervention, we find that reduction is everything that implies *reducing the measure of a factor* with actions leading to the original state or closest to it.

It should be mentioned that Harm Reduction differs from Risk Reduction, since the first is to avoid as much as possible the negative effects due to the use of substances, i.e., it pretends to reduce the harmful aspects that such practice may cause, promoting healthy and hygienic habits, so that the drug abusers will have an active participation in the event of consumption and their habits regarding such consumption. While the second term becomes an educational-health activity involving the problem regarding the consequences of drug abuse and the main population targeted is the one with no treatment related with its consumption [43].

The program for the patient with alcohol consumption started in 1974 at the Hospital General de México and in 1982 with the first Anti-Smoking Clinic (CCT), the latter program, ahead of their age, carried out multidisciplinary protocols addressed to the prevention, early and timely detection of diseases consequence of tobacco consumption, where therapeutic adherence played a very important role for the rehabilitation of the patient, as well as health education programs that will allow users know from their addiction to nicotine to their physical illness, in addition to a whole range of activities that will allow them modify their thoughts, behaviors and emotions that surround the consumption of the substance, achieving through this model the reduction of the damages [30]. The research carried out at the General Hospital of Mexico in which it compares two therapeutic techniques: cognitive restructuring and health education; the cessation obtained with the first was 52% while the second was 56%, important results because they indicate that by only applying health education the person can reach the cessation of the use of psychoactive substances [44].

In 2015 the treatment focused on all psychoactive substances, since the changes of the time were observed in the lifestyles of the population attending the anti-smoking clinic, because of which, from 2000 to 2010, 934 patients were studied demonstrating that 47% of users used more than one drug. Likewise, the inadequate processes were investigated in lifestyles where uncontrolled intake of soda and coffee was found between 64.1 and 68.4% [45] and sedentary life 61.8%. Other studies in this population also showed low level of assertiveness and social skills deficit [46]. Given these findings, the proposal is made through a holistic approach with the sum of the different medical specialties and subspecialties for the comorbidities by apparatus and system, as well as the psychological intervention, to abandon the different consumptions of psychoactive substances, widening their field of attention, monitoring the medical guidelines with therapeutic adherence, with a psychoeducational and active orientation in which it is intended to generate, strengthen and use the protective factors of each individual with therapies based on learning theories for the recovery of their physical and mental health and creating an intervention where the priority is still to reduce harm.

In the anti-smoking and other addictive substances clinics, the objective is for medical personnel to resume their activity in adherence to treatment as a fundamental tool for their work versus psychologists who are involved in the recovery and compliance of the treatment of medical or psychiatric comorbidities and not only work with cessation. Since we can observe that intrinsically the most important were bad habits in lifestyles, the discipline in self-care is responsible for playing a good role in their health and their execution is responsible for not consuming substances. Thus, within Harm Reduction Intervention proposed in a comprehensive care model, adherence to treatment has an important weight in the recovery of the person with substance abuse.

6. Adherence to treatment

Adherence to treatment allows patient to have greater control over chronic degenerative diseases. Commitment of patients, along with their motivation, is essential to continue such treatment, since it is relatively complex, prolonged and requires discipline, planning and adaptation to change. Chronic complications related to the use of psychoactive substances or drugs can be avoided or delayed if the person follows the instructions given by health specialists. The treatment that patients with dependence receive focuses on the modification of addictive behaviors but unfortunately poor adherence is a very common situation and the high dropout rate is one of the factors that generate the greatest concern in the consumption of drugs [47].

The World Health Organization conducted an investigation to determine the level of adherence to treatment of people with chronic diseases living in developed countries. The results indicated that about only 50% of the people followed the indications and assumed that this deficiency would be greater in developing countries (such as Mexico) due to the scarcity of resources and inequities in access to medical care a fact still present nowadays [48].

The WHO [48] considers the lack of adherence to treatments and its negative clinical and economic consequences a priority public health issue. It also considers that compliance with treatments will result in a reduction of the overall health budget, due to the reduction in the need for expensive interventions, such as frequent and prolonged hospitalizations, the unnecessary use of emergency services and costly intensive care services. If patients fail to have a good adherence, they will have great losses at a personal (physical and psychological), family and social level. In the United States, for example, poor adherence to taking the medication is related to 33–69% of hospitalizations [49]. An important point is that once again, the social determinants of health play an important role in allowing patients to adhere to their treatment, as well as on their socioeconomic status, public policies regarding social protection or the structure of the health system where they belong.

There are different definitions of adherence to treatment, one of the definitions that has been most widely accepted and which the WHO resumed in 2003 is the one proposed by Haynes [50] who defines it as "the degree to which a patient's behavior in relation to taking medications, following a diet or changing lifestyle habits, coincides with the instructions provided by the doctor or healthcare staff." It can be said that there is adherence when patients collaborate and participate proactively and voluntarily with their treatment, promoting better health conditions, which go beyond passive compliance with the indications [51].

Adherence is influenced by several psychosocial factors, such as beliefs, attitudes, attributions, mental representation of the disease and social support [52, 53]. Adherence as a health behavior will be closely related to the general health values or motivation for health, it will also be modulated by the experimentation of risk or perceived vulnerability, the consideration of the severity of the disease and self-efficacy [54] (**Figure 2**).

For the consumers to change their lifestyle, they first need to modify their belief system, since this is an important modulating factor in compliance with medical and/or health recommendations. The person follows the indications based on the considerations of his/her personal beliefs and on the perception of the origin of his/her illness or the way he/she thinks he/she should face his/her health condition [55]. Patients have a representation of what a threat to their health means, their fears are concepts based on social learning in their relationships with others [56]. There are several sources that influence beliefs about their health: friends, family, media and information from other health professionals [57]. Patient beliefs regarding the treatment produce and maintain healthy behaviors. The specialist has to establish realistic expectations about the benefits patients will get when changing their lifestyle but take into consideration the time and effort required.

A strategic source of adherence to treatment is assertive communication, which occurs between the patient with addiction and the specialist. During the communication exercise presented during the first approaches, especially during the first interview, it is essential to identify the level of predisposition that the person has to modify his/her addictive behavior. This level is directly related to the degree

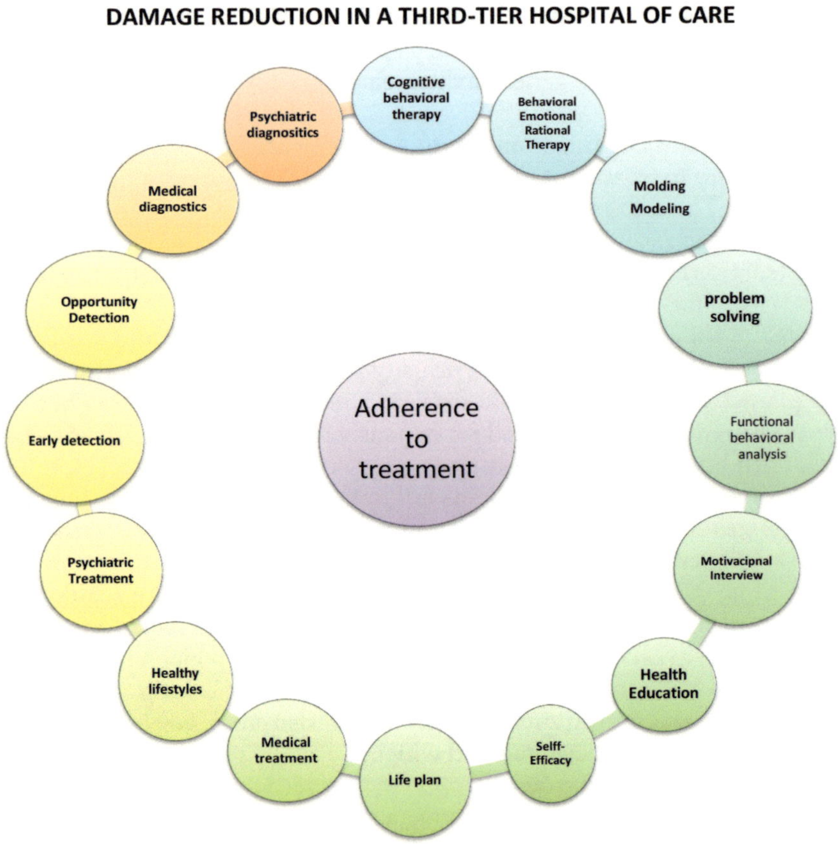

Figure 2.
The treatment is directed towards the prevention of physical and psychiatric risk factors through a multidisciplinary intervention with the intervention of psychology, psychiatry and the different medical specialties [47].

of motivation of a patient, since it predicts whether consumption will remain the same or will change favorably [58]. To recognize and work on the motivation to change, the Transteoric Change Model and the Motivational Interview formulated by Prochaska and DiClemente [59] stand out in order to identify different levels of predisposition that a person can show *-stages of change-* when it is proposed to modify his/her addictive behavior [60]. Thus, favoring respect for the patient, his/her beliefs and scale of values, trying to stimulate his/her motivation and favor his/her positioning towards healthy habits, emphasizing his/her own point of view and his/her freedom to choose. Progressively increasing the willingness to change, becoming aware of the problem and developing the necessary strategies to overcome it, including the skills to overcome contingencies and relapse. To go through the process of motivation to change in a stable and constant way, promoting his/her level of self-efficacy and allowing him/her to have greater adherence. Besides, by emphasizing the discovery of his/her risk factors we will also work on protective factors, since both have a relevant role during the onset, development, maintenance and treatment of addictions [59].

7. Conclusion

In order to globally address the consumption of psychoactive substances, the clinical history is the indispensable information tool that will establish the meeting point with precision and the scientific, ethical, technological criteria that will be included in it, through their participation in its preparation between the different health professionals [61]. The integration will generate a unique file resulting in comprehensive management and attention, which serves as an effective communication meeting point for the treatment and evolution of the disciplines that converge, as well as the homogenization of decision-making subsequent to the diagnosis established by the consumption of legal and illegal substances, and will influence with good practices on the diagnosis, treatment, rehabilitation, of the "drug" abusers and achieve healthy lifestyles, with the priority of enriching his/her quality of life, decreasing the risks, as well as motivating the user as far as possible to eradicate substance abuse through techniques for restructuring his/her beliefs, behaviors and emotions. Besides, the health professional will accept, in a more committed way, that the consumer may feel worried about his/her health even if he/she does not succeed or does not want to stop its consumption.

Finally, the first thing to conceive in the field of health, what we have been working on for decades, is to state that the harm reduction intervention focuses on the tertiary prevention framework, which is carried out once the problem has appeared and its objective is to avoid complications, reducing risks [62], transcending in the general improvement of patients (adherence to treatment/self-efficacy, self-care) and increasing their physical and psychological recovery by encouraging abstinence and preventing relapses; reaching an approach that achieves the integral health of the users with interdisciplinary interventions, reducing the cost and increasing the benefit for the hospital users and their families, as well as for the psychological institution, reducing the cost and increasing the benefit for the hospital users and their families as well as for the institution.

Author details

María Angélica Ocampo*, César Guillermo Popoca, Abraham Sánchez, Catalina Casillas and Raúl Cicero
"Dr. Eduardo Liceaga" General Hospital of Mexico, Mexico

*Address all correspondence to: ccthgmod@yahoo.com.mx; magnetowilde@gmail.com

References

[1] NIDA. Drugs, Brains, and Behavior: The Science of Addiction. National Institute on Drug Abuse. 2018. Available from: https://www.drugabuse.gov/publications/drugs-brains-behavior-science-addiction

[2] American Psychiatric Association (APA). Diagnostic and Statistical Manual of Mental Disorders (DSM-5). 5th ed. Washington, DC: American Psychiatric Association; 2013

[3] Wu E et al. The association between substance use and intimate partner violence within black male same-sex relationships. Journal of Interpersonal Violence. 2015;**30**(5):762-781

[4] Magis-Rodríguez C, García-Sánchez JA, Marín-Navarrete R. Harm reduction among people who inject drugs in Mexico. Salud Mental. 2018;**41**(4):153-156

[5] Institute for Health Metrics and Evaluation. Findings from the Global Burden of Disease Study. Seattle: IHME; 2018. Available from: http://www.healthdata.org/policy-report/findings-global-burden-disease-study-2017

[6] United Nations Office on Drugs and Crime. Executive Summary Conclusions and Policy Implications. Vienna: WHO; 2019. Available from: https://wdr.unodc.org/wdr2019/index.html

[7] United Nations Office on Drugs and Crime. Executive Summary Conclusions and Policy Implications. Vienna: WHO; 2018. Available from: https://www.unodc.org/wdr2018/

[8] World Health Organization. WHO Framework Convention on Tobacco Control: Guidelines for Implementation of Article 5. 3, Articles 8 To 14. Geneva: World Health Organization; 2013. Available from: https://www.who.int/fctc/treaty_instruments/adopted/guidel_2011/en/

[9] World Health Organization. Global Status Report on Alcohol and Health. Geneva: World Health Organization; 2018. Available from: https://www.who.int/substance_abuse/publications/global_alcohol_report/en/

[10] Inter-American Drug Abuse Control Commission (CICAD). Report on Drug Use in the Americas. Washington: Organization of American States; 2019. Available from: http://cicad.oas.org/Main/ssMain/E-report_ENG_2019/mobile/index.html

[11] Drug Enforcement Administration (DEA). National Drug Threat Assessment. United States: U.S. Department of Justice; 2018. Available from: https://www.dea.gov/press-releases/2018/11/02/dea-releases-2018-national-drug-threat-assessment-0

[12] Ramón de la Fuente Muñiz National Institute of Psychiatry. National Survey on Drug, Alcohol and Tobacco Use, ENCODAT 2016-2017. México: Secretariat of Health; 2017. Available from: https://www.gob.mx/salud%7Cconadic/acciones-y-programas/encuesta-nacional-de-consumo-de-drogas-alcohol-y-tabaco-encodat-2016-2017-136758

[13] CONADIC. CONADIC Presents Preventive Guidelines for Children, Adolescents, Parents and Teachers; 2017. Available from: https://www.gob.mx/salud/conadic/acciones-y-programas/conadic-presenta-guias-preventivas-para-ninos-ninas-adolescentes-padres-y-maestros-108566

[14] National Commission Against Addiction (CONADIC). Report on the Situation of Drug Use in Mexico and Its Comprehensive Care. Ciudad de

México: Secretariat of Health; 2019. Available from: https://www.gob.mx/salud/conadic/documentos/informe-sobre-la-situacion-de-las-drogas-en-mexico-y-su-atencion-integral-2019

[15] Alejandra MS, Páez HJV. Sostenibilidad del Gasto Público: cobertura y financiamiento de enfermedades crónicas en México. Ensayos Revista de Economía. 2018;**37**(1):99-133

[16] Pan American Health Organization. Health in the Americas+, 2017 Edition. Summary: Regional Outlook and Country Profiles. PAHO: Washington, D.C; 2017. Available from: http://iris.paho.org/xmlui/handle/123456789/34321

[17] Urbina-Fuentes M et al. Transition from millennium development goals to sustainable development goals from the perspective of the social determinants of health and health equity. Gaceta Médica de México. 2017;**153**(6):697-730

[18] National Council for the Evaluation of Social Development Policy (CONEVAL). Ten Years of Measuring Multidimensional Poverty in Mexico: Advances and Challenges in Social Policy Measuring Poverty 2008-2018. Ciudad de México: CONEVAL; 2019. Available from: https://www.coneval.org.mx/SalaPrensa/Comunicadosprensa/Documents/2019/COMUNICADO_10_MEDICION_POBREZA_2008_2018.pdf

[19] Valdés H. Análisis crítico del rol del Estado frente a los derechos sociales y en particular el derecho a la salud. Santiago, Chile: Universidad de Chile - Facultad de Derecho; 2018. Available from: http://repositorio.uchile.cl/handle/2250/152795

[20] Medina FIA et al. Perfil clínico y metabólico de la persona con diabetes tipo 2 en control ambulatorio de Oxkutzcab, Yucatán. Revista de Estudios Clínicos e Investigación Psicológica. 2017;**7**(14):58-69

[21] World Health Organization [Internet]. Geneva: Social Determinants of Health. 2019. Available from: https://www.who.int/social_determinants/en/

[22] Church AT. Personality traits across cultures. Current Opinion in Psychology. 2016;**8**:22-30. DOI: 10.1016/j.copsyc.2015.09.014

[23] Scott E. Reinforcement principles for addiction medicine; from recreational drug use to psychiatric disorder. In: Waxman S, Stein DG, Swaab D, Fields H, editors. Progress in Brain Resea. London: Elsevier; 2016. pp. 63-76

[24] Glyn D et al. The role of lifestyle in perpetuating substance use disorder: the lifestyle balance model. Substance Abuse Treatment, Prevention, and Policy. 2015;**10**(1):2

[25] Bandura A, Riviere A. Social Learning Theory. Madrid: Espasa-calpe; 1984

[26] Grekin GC. Manejo de la obesidad a través de un programa multidisciplinario. Ars Medica [internet]. 1997;**26**(1). [cited 09 October 2020] [aprox. 12p]. Available from: https://doi.org/10.11565/arsmed.v26i1.1208

[27] Montesinos J, Guerri C. Consecuencias neuropatológicas y conductuales del abuso de alcohol durante la adolescencia. In: Martínez TL, editor. Consumo de alcohol en jóvenes y adolescentes. Una mirada ecológica, 30. Bilbao: Universidad de Deusto; 2014. Available from: https://dialnet.unirioja.es/servlet/articulo?codigo=6998264

[28] Sanz MM. Epigenética y trastornos psiquiátricos. Pediatría Integral. 2015;**19**(8):524. Available from: https://

www.pediatriaintegral.es/wp-content/uploads/2015/12/Pediatria-Integral-XIX-8_WEB.pdf#page=8

[29] Armando A-LA. Revisión y análisis sobre la efectividad del modelo multidisciplinario para la atención de la diabetes. Horizonte Sanitario. 2019;**18**(3). Available from: file:///C:/Users/CARDIO~1/AppData/Local/Temp/3300-18032-1-PB.pdf

[30] Ocampo MA. Proposal for the transition from the anti-smoking clinic to the day care clinic for tobacco, alcohol, addictive behaviors and other drugs at the General Hospital of Mexico O. D [Master's thesis]. Postgraduate Center of the State of Mexico (CPEM); 2011

[31] Marlatt GA. Prevención de recaídas en conductas adictivas basada en Mindfulness. Desclée de Brouwer; 2013

[32] Míguez MDC. Los procedimientos de autoayuda para dejar de fumar. Monografía Tabaco. 2004;**16**(suplemento 2):339

[33] Schwartz JL. Review and Evaluation of Smoking Cessation Methods: The United States and Canada, 1978-1985. Washington, DC: U.S. Department of Health and Human Services; 1987

[34] Becoña I. El tratamiento psicológico de la adicción a la nicotina. Papeles del Psicólogo. 2003;**24**(85):48-69

[35] Sanz J et al. El tratamiento del tabaquismo en los entros de Drogodependencias y Unidades de Conductas Adictivas. Adicciones. 2004;**16**(Suppl 2):321-337

[36] Sterling S, Chi F, Hinman A. Integrating care for people with co-occurring alcohol and other drug, medical, and mental health conditions. Alcohol Research & Health. 2011;**33**(4):338-349

[37] Savic M, Best D, Manning V, et al. Strategies to facilitate integrated care for people with alcohol and other drug problems: A systematic review. Substance Abuse Treatment, Prevention, and Policy. 2017;**12**:19

[38] Bosque-Prous M, Brugal MT. Harm reduction interventions in drug users: Current situation and recommendations. Gaceta Sanitaria. 2016;**30**:99-105

[39] Tizoc-Marquez A et al. Reduction of damage as a strategy for the use and abuse of substances in Mexico: Challenges and opportunities. Ra Ximhai. 2017;**13**(2):39-51

[40] Velázquez Benítez D, Friman Rodríguez N, González García M. Addiction damage reduction programs, an ethical dilemma. Medical Scientific Mail of Holguín. 2016;**20**(4):804-809

[41] Harm Reduction International (HRI). The Global State of Harm Reduction. London: HRI; 2016. Available from: https://www.hri.global/contents/1739

[42] Corominas J. Breve diccionario etimológico de la lengua castellana 3ra Ed. Madrid: Gredos; 1967

[43] Casado Gallego J. Consumo responsable de sustancias: La reducción de riesgos como alternativa a la prohibición; 2013

[44] Ocampo MA. Smoking Cessation Program in a Third Level Hospital. CONADIC: México; 2007. Available from: http://148.204.52.13/i/bibliotecaDase/2000/Acervo/AcervoVirtualSalud/SaludAcervoLecturas/Terapia.pdf

[45] Ocampo MA, Cicero-Sabido R. Retos de la medicina actual: Los 30 años de experiencia de la clínica contra

el tabaco del Hospital General de México "Dr. Eduardo Liceaga". Revista Médica del Hospital General de México. 2012;**75**(3):180-184

[46] Leal BM, Ocampo MA, Cicero R. Niveles de asertividad, perfil sociodemográfico, dependencia a la nicotina y motivos para fumar en una población de fumadores que acude a un tratamiento para dejar de fumar. Salud Mental. 2010;**33**(6):489-497

[47] García FC, Costa J, Piquer RV. Motivos de abandono temprano de pacientes en tratamiento ambulatorio de adicción a sustancias. Revista Española de Drogodependencias. 2016;**1**(1):41-55

[48] World Health Organization (WHO) Adherence to Long-Term Therapies. Evidence for Action. Geneva: WHO; 2003. Available from: https://www.who.int/chp/knowledge/publications/adherence_full_report.pdf?ua=1

[49] Oung AB, Kosirog E, Chavez B, Brunner J, Saseen JJ. Evaluation of medication adherence in chronic disease at a federally qualified health center. Therapeutic Advances in Chronic Disease. 2016;**8**(8-9):113-120

[50] Hayness RB, Taylor DW, Sackett DL, editors. Compliance in Health Care. Baltimore, MD: Johns Hopkins University Press; 1979. p. 516

[51] López-Romero LA, Romero-Guevara SL, Parra DI, Rojas-Sánchez LZ. Adherencia al tratamiento: Concepto y medición. Revista Hacia la Promoción de la Salud. 2016;**21**(1):117-137

[52] Pedraza Banderas GL, Vega Valero CZ. Caracterización psicosocial de pacientes diabéticos mexicanos. Revista Electrónica de Psicología Iztacala. 2019;**21**(4):1371-1393

[53] Puente Silva FG. What Is Therapeutic Adherence? Therapeutic Adhesion. Implications for Mexico. 1st ed. Consejo Regional Latinoamericano y del Caribe de Salud Mental: México; 1985

[54] Ramos Morales LE. Adherence to treatment in chronic diseases. Journal of Angiology & Vascular Surgery. 2015;**16**(2):175-189

[55] Pérez Rosabal E, Sánchez S, María Y, Morales Ortiz L. Adherencia terapéutica y creencias sobre su salud en pacientes hipertensos. MediSan. 2016;**20**(1):3-9

[56] Bandura A. Psychological Modeling: Conflicting Theories. New York: Routledge; 2017

[57] Ocampo A, Hernández TE, Sabido RC. Consumption of psychoactive substances in hospitalized patients in the pneumology service of a third-level general hospital. Journal of Substance Use. 2018;**23**(5):481-484

[58] Usurin G, Cindy M, Isacupe M, Milagros K. Effectiveness of Motivational Interview to Improve Treatment in People with Addiction to Psychoactive Substances [Grade of Specialty]. Lima, Peru: Norbert Wienerfacultad Private University of Health Sciences; 2019. Available from: http://repositorio.uwiener.edu.pe/handle/123456789/3017

[59] Hashemzadeh M, Rahimi A, Zare-Farashbandi F, Alavi-Naeini AM, Daei A. Transtheoretical model of health behavioral change: A systematic review. Iranian Journal of Nursing and Midwifery Research. 2019;**24**(2):83-90

[60] Ocampo MA. The role of healthcare professionals in tobacco care. In: Medina-Mora ME, editor. Smoking in Mexico How to Avoid 60,000 Premature Deaths Every Year? México: El Colegio Nacional; 2010. p. 744

[61] NOM-004-SSA3-2012 [en línea]. México: National Consultative Committee for Standardization of Innovation, Development, Technologies and Health Information; 2012. Available from: http://sitios.dif.gob.mx/normateca/disposiciones-generales/normas-oficiales/

[62] Becoña E. Bases científicas de la prevención de las drogadicciones. 1st ed. Madrid: Ministerio del Interior; 2002